BRØKEN &
JUST AS SWEET

The Amazing Grace of Motherhood, Marriage, and Miracles on the Spectrum

Marisa Ulrich

eLectio Publishing

Little Elm, TX

www.eLectioPublishing.com

Broken Cookies Taste Just as Sweet: The Amazing Grace of Motherhood, Marriage, and Miracles on the Spectrum
By Marisa Ulrich

Copyright 2016 by Marisa Ulrich
Cover Design by eLectio Publishing

ISBN-13: 978-1-63213-138-6
Published by eLectio Publishing, LLC
Little Elm, Texas
http://www.eLectioPublishing.com

Printed in the United States of America

5 4 3 2 1 eLP 21 20 19 18 17 16

The eLectio Publishing editing team is comprised of: Christine LePorte, Lori Draft, Sheldon James, Court Dudek, Kaitlyn Campbell, and Jim Eccles.

Publisher's Note
The publisher does not have any control over and does not assume any responsibility for author or third-party websites or their content.

Dedicated to any who have encouraged us along the way.
You each have your part.

And to my dear Joseph,
who never let this book fall victim to the dreaded delete button.

CONTENTS

Chapter One

Introductions, Introspections, and the Like

Let's begin with what this book is not. It's not how to raise autistic children. It's not how to raise so-called typical children. It's not how to be married to someone who is unofficially on the spectrum as one who is not—officially. (I didn't walk away without a single trait, honestly. I am yet examining myself as my children become more and more a mirror back into my own experiences.)

It's not even how *not* to lose your mind in the process of bringing this all together.

It's not a tragedy, though I have cried a bushel of buckets in these years.

It's not a comedy, though there has been room for belly laughs enough for a dozen *Carol Burnett Shows*.

It's well…it's just life, okay?

I don't have ten steps for making your days run smoother. I don't have the seven keys to successful breakthrough. This isn't trendy motivational schtick, life-changing therapy, or an instruction manual.

Definitely not a pep talk, is it?

There are times in our lives when we may need such answers. Darned if I'm the one to provide them, though.

For, you see, my answers have been found in my biggest, most face-flattening stumbles. I have found the greatest triumphs in my life through the trip-ups and hiccups. Much as I want to appear sleek and worldly-wise to you, I am still very much a shy, dorky, incredibly insecure twelve-year-old trapped in this aging lady's body.

I must surrender dreams of poise and listen to the Father, who urges me on lovingly.

Pssst, Marisa! The mess! He says. *The mess!* Not *the success!*

"The mess? The ugly, stinky, pooey, awful mess?!" I whine to my Lord. "Whyyyy?"

Well, His eternally patient reply, bending down from Heaven to tuck my hair behind my ear with a daddy's love, *the mess is where the* miracles *happen, my dear.*

Yes, too true, I must acknowledge. Oh, not merely miracles such as splitting a large body of water from top to toe or popping a piece of gold out of a flounder's floppy kisser, though some things have hit us about the same way as a sudden fish slap.

Those are great, and I am antsy as a three-year-old waiting to meet Elmo to relate them to you. And I will.

But I also aim to share those things we might forget to appreciate until we have a life crumbled to a crisp then raised from curling, smoking ash.

Until you find your child doesn't match the charts. Or the pigeonholes. Or any other category people in this life want to squeeze us into. And somehow, he finds his way.

Until you have had your high school sweetheart say, "Catch ya later!" to start family two while family one consists of mommy, toddler, baby, and waiting-to-debut. And somehow, you pick up and walk on.

Until you have had to swing time off for a dozen tests, a leaning tower of paperwork, and three IEP meetings in one year on a single mother's small salary and crazy schedule. And somehow, it all gets done.

Until you have had every sincere-sounding guy run for the hills when you say the words autism spectrum disorder. Or three kids. Or I love Jesus. And then…someone doesn't run.

Until you have had those bills whose numbers mirror national debt to pay like *now* and have only a mama dollar and papa dollar to your name. And somehow, they get paid.

The miracles of getting through. Getting better. Getting progress. Those are miracles as much as those testimonies of the instant rise from a deathbed or angelic intervention on a slick, frozen highway.

We just don't always seem to see them. Because they're, well, they're life. They roll out almost in automatic fashion with sometimes scarcely a nod from us.

I don't say it is exclusive to folks like me, but there is such a joy you never know until you have begun the process of raising special needs children. Every moment of overcoming, be it tolerating loud hand dryers without tears, crossing a bridge without fear of falling through the cracks, buttoning pants without a hitch...every little thing so taken for granted becomes huge.

Worthy of claps, whoops, and celebratory dance.

And yes, that also, at times, makes the disappointments huge, too, even if they might seem minor to others. The wondering if they'll ever get it, or is this it? Will the rest of your life be taken up by helping your nine-year-old daughter tip her head back in the shower so the water doesn't scare her so badly she can't shampoo? Setbacks and stagnation can be hard to tackle on any given day.

That's when you go to the Father, again and again, to lay it down and take up a new dose of His endless grace. You cry. And then you help rinse her hair. Because she's yours. And you love her. And there's no one like her.

Those are the sorts of things I want to tell you about, every bit as much as those wow moments that have made up this life of mine in the spectrum sandwich. The mess that somehow always proceeds the miracle....

Confession. I never really dreamt of motherhood. As per older brother/main mentor's instructions—go figure!—my dolls were all gangs of boys instead of helpless babes for me to coddle and coo to. I wouldn't have known where to begin on diapering and bottle-feeding.

And mothers seemed so tired. Thankless. Ever elusive and ever angry with the likes of shy, clumsy me.

I felt I couldn't please her to save my life. What would ever possess me to presume I could do her job when I had failed so miserably to succeed at even the task of childhood?

And for a good five years into my first marriage, it looked like God agreed motherhood was not in my wheelhouse. Working with kids others had produced and sweated through sleepless nights with seemed to be more in line with my calling.

I could love on them a little, understand their foibles and follies, and send them on their way without the frightening investment of giving birth and raising them to adulthood.

And then, all of a sudden, there he was, right in my belly, crowding into my insecure life. Elijah Richard.

And all of a sudden, I had the daunting task of trying to learn what it was to pour myself into a tiny, fragile being.

We stumbled, and we tottered, and we came through that first year or so all right, though not without much weeping and frustration.

And then, when he was around two or so, I began to observe there was something rather uncommon in my little boy.

I think it began with *Blue's Clues*.

Every child has their fair amount of obsessions. This I know after years of teaching preschool. But Elijah's was, well, different.

He could be mesmerized by that little blue puppy to the extent of dismissing all else around him. Soon, he was drawing clues in

4

his own Handy Dandy Notebook, his scrawls not so much childish as uncanny matches for what was on the screen. Then, he was memorizing chunks—whole episodes—and spouting them off verbatim.

Genius? Cute parlor trick? Not so much.

You see, all this was coming at the exclusion of almost any other conversation, any other pursuit.

Except, perhaps, the climbing.

In his eyes, everything in our small apartment was worth scaling from entertainment center to shelves to refrigerator. The latter he perched atop long enough to draw a circle on the ceiling I couldn't reach to clean.

Yes, I know. Tssk, tssk, neglectful mommy.

I won't excuse myself under the umbrella of postpartum depression, but unless you have experienced its gripping fear and self-loathing, you can't know how each day is such a hill to climb.

A tired sort of anxiety had overtaken my rather isolated existence, and with a husband who was often more absent than present and a spiritual life more depleted than complete, the aloneness reared up that much larger in my eyes.

Anyway...needless to say, Elijah was an unusual sort of fellow. Busy beyond the norm, difficult to manage, often caught up in a world that seemed to appeal on a level Mom, Dad, and peers did not.

I first explored the possibilities in an online search. Time and again, autism rose up on the screen before me. Difficult to consider, yet difficult to deny.

Would that someone had given me more than a perfunctory ear in that time. Yet there was such an all-around dismissal and false reassurance that his words would come and toddlerhood drive would fade, and rightly or wrongly, I found myself acquiescing and laying the anxieties aside—at least out loud.

Within, however, the questions had their fruitless field day.

And into this atmosphere came a second boy. Timothy Joel. Two weeks behind schedule. Labor induced, rescued from my womb in the wee hours by emergency C-section when his heart didn't tolerate the inducement. Revived from his very still blue state when he inhaled meconium on the trip out. Eight days as the biggest baby the NICU had, hands stiff and adorned with tiny braces to force the thumbs out of his tight little fists.

Upon his homecoming, there were equal parts fanfare and apprehension. As a result of his thumbs, occupational therapy visits in the home were prescribed. This was my first encounter with such outside help. I was both excited to see what might be accomplished and nervous I'd be outed as the fraud of a mother I so often felt I was.

Where Timothy was concerned, I found I needn't have fretted much. He excelled in gripping the things they wished for him to grip and tested out three months ahead of schedule. This was sort of a prelude to the determination to succeed that always seemed to propel the little guy.

Elijah, on the other hand, displayed those baffling behaviors for every therapist and special needs worker to see. At Timothy's IEP meeting, he sidled right up to one gentleman and greeted him with his best *Blue's Clues* then fell into the incomprehensible tongue we could only term "Elijahspeak." It sounded like a cross between Japanese and alien.

I was urged to keep a close eye on his speech development. If this sort of communication was still the norm by age three, testing would be the next recommendation.

I nodded my head and tucked this disturbing yet utterly unsurprising news in my head with the rest of my fears and kept on stepping as best I could.

Still without much support despite now having expert opinions on my side. Not to disparage my family by any means.

Perhaps we were all in some manner or form of denial or blind hope.

Or further distracted by two events that fell one atop the other.

Just as Elijah rounded the corner to three in February, behavior and speech not much improved, I found myself once again surprised by impending motherhood. I can admit to weariness and a scrambling to reconcile my much-weighted fate.

By April's end, my eyes were opened to another surprise. This one struck squarely between the eyes.

My husband of eight years was in love with another woman.

He had met her while she was in his employ. The strains of home, loss of direction, and lack of communication so inherent to us both contributed to the downfall. I can't say I knew it then, but I know enough now to say confidently that I cannot lay his choices at my feet nor punish myself because of them.

By May, his bags were packed, and though it was denied at the outset, he quickly set up residence with the new love of his life.

My self-esteem in rags, I chose this time to wake my sleeping sense of marital duty, praying with all my might reconciliation might be possible. But this latent sacrifice on my part was of little avail. His mind and heart were set, though there were many lofty promises of remaining an active father.

Suicide began to tug at me as it had in depressions past from childhood onward. I came dangerously near the self-destruct button. It was the wake-up call of three little lives dependent upon me, one still awaiting her big debut, that really shook it out of me.

It was hard to find the joy of living, of course, at this time. I found myself full-out on the altar, again and again, seeking God's face as well as the strength and grace to face another day.

And almost before I knew it, that first summer of aloneness, of storms within and without, drew to a close. October chilled the

Kansas air, and our one and only daughter, Sarah Elisabeth, came to soothe my restless aching world.

To his credit, her father was present for the birth, though his exit after was swift, unsaid demands of the new woman replacing the old.

It was a long night in the darkness of that hospital room, wakeful and busy in caring for this precious girl on my own while my boys rested in the comfort of Grandpa and Grandma's arms. Dear brother was there, too, working at getting on his feet after physical setbacks, yet still finding time to teach Elijah to write his name, love on Timbo, admire Sarah, and keep me boosted through this new phase.

Funny how this home full of memories both good and terrible had become our go-to place, the devastation of our existence in those days unexpectedly threading us tighter together. Love tends to bloom as reliance grows. The abuses of times past faded to forgiveness in the unadulterated need of each other. Healing *had* begun many years before this sudden turn, but somehow the very bittersweet of these days sealed the fact for us.

We were family, for better or worse. And we were sticking together.

And so we settled into a new normal, with much prayer and faith-expanding occurring along the way. I continued to seek His face in earnest, His covering for the sometimes howling pain. The Word came to life in a way it hadn't since my avid teen years. In between running after babies and toddler, I snatched every morsel I could.

I was financially able via the state to stay home that first year. Say what you might about assistance, but I will be forever grateful.

The children and I bumped along in those early days of just the four of us, baby Sarah a lovely little novelty. Her sweetness proved a vastly wonderful consolation prize, a salve to so many tearful days.

Timothy quickly left babyhood behind in exchange for older brother, and Elijah began to string together a few more phrases, but the pressing need to intervene in the odd course of his young life continued to haunt.

When the time drew near for Sarah's first birthday, my mind was made up. The state's generous assistance would begin to scale back, child support was an inconsistent pittance, and the prospect of becoming a working mom loomed.

As terrified as I was, I would waste no time. I began scouring the want ads. Not many days passed before an ad for a daycare teacher popped out to me. A place of work I knew well, and a potential launch from which to finally settle what the difference was with my Elijah, who was months away from five with limping progress at best.

The name of the school was Trinity, a hopeful sign of God's direction to come. Almost before I could turn around, this longtime single mom's first interview promised employment.

And so the years of home and four gray walls reminding me of singleness were left behind. The working mama years had commenced…

Chapter Two
Testing, Testing…
One, Two, Three

I plunged into teaching with a fair amount of trepidation. Those early weeks were filled with missteps, exhaustion, and a heavy sense of longing for my babies, who were back at home with my mother.

Most people were kind, patient, and accommodating as I struggled to find my feet, my voice, my niche. It was clear I was still attempting to surmount the deep grief of losing my marriage and my way of life, and while I strived to be the hard worker I always determined to be, it was also evident I was floundering, the unsure shades of the abused child in me causing needed firmness with my students to crumble.

Thankfully, my boss must've seen more in me than I could at the time. With some strategic trading of classrooms, I began to settle in with a smaller, more manageable brood and gain a measure of confidence I had not felt in myself in so very long.

And then, at last, the door opened for Elijah to attend the four and five-year-old class. My intentions to get him tested were well-known from the get-go.

I also attempted to prepare his teachers for the dawn-to-dusk tornado he could be, to translate his most obscure phrases, and advocate for some of the stranger behaviors.

But frankly, nothing truly prepares a teacher inexperienced with autism for what it really can be like to spend a school day with it.

There was a lot of frustration all the way around for a time, honestly. I was much the mother hen, and they were much the put-upon educators. And coworkers to boot.

Needless to say, it was not the smoothest of transitions. But to their credit, his teachers survived, as did their heads from the hair-pulling.

And though there were days I honestly went home quietly angry—and days I came back not so quietly angry—I survived as well.

And learned much about how to defend my child properly and politely.

And Elijah? Well, he went on his merry way most days, doing his own thing with very little concern for how he was perceived. Yet into all this I began to see something else being woven in on other days. A desire to belong, at least a little. A response that brought about a modicum of friendship in some and, sadly, a thirst for bullying in others.

There was a time or two of rescuing him from dogpiles in those early days. Something a parent never dreams of having to do for her child.

Yet I found in myself a gratefulness to God I was there to do so. Sometimes, I suppose, as obnoxious as we are on other fronts, there is a use for us mother hens. :)

About this time, the initial round of papers and testing was begun to determine what his needs might be.

We met so many people in those days, from social workers to behavioral, occupational, physical, and speech therapists to people whose sole job was to mesh findings and measure against criteria.

It was lovely to hear time and again from people who were taken with him, had actually *seen* kids like him, and seemed to have some clue about where to go from there, even if they didn't have all the immediate answers I hoped for. Something I soon discovered was that autism is a long road, and there are many stops before and after it is finally pinpointed.

So…after mountains of paperwork, one test after another, many missed work hours—*Thanks, boss! You were awesome!*—one conclusion was easily reached. Elijah was smart as a whip in rote skills but behind his peers in his speech, motor skills, and behavior. But to diagnose him firmly? Well, apparently, in his case, it was too soon. He was too young. I can admit it was frustrating at times to still have no diagnosis in hand, to be halted a bit on the road, and to hear, *Yeah, he's behind, and autism is probably why, but where he fits on this huge spectrum, who knows?*

He did, thankfully, qualify for some care—from behavioral to motor skills to speech—and they began to hook him up with great therapists who tackled the process of deciphering what "I go home cheeseburger" meant (as clear as it sounds—I'm done with you people, and I want to go home and have my favorite meal) as well as more challenging things such as why you should not try to free the goldfish from the comfy confines of its bowl, tear apart the decorative blow-up animal your mommy's boss put up to celebrate Rodeo Days, or allow a pack of boys to dogpile you on the playground. Some days were better than others, obviously, and there was much learning to go around for student and teachers alike.

I won't lie. It was rather refreshing to see the educating happening on both sides.

Elijah continued to be a rarity in his classroom and in the daycare in general. He was a guinea pig, so to speak.

Though not the first in the daycare's long history to have needs beyond the norm, he certainly remained a unique challenge.

And then, amazingly, marvelous affection grew.

For him.

From him.

It was a short tenure he spent in their care, really. But in that time, with therapy a helpful building block, startling things began to happen.

He began to unfurl some of those long dormant things inside and experience growth.

When he started attending, his sentences were four words long at best, but when he left eight months later, he was kindergarten ready, with a few accommodations, and best of all, talking a blue streak. And not just about *Blue's Clues*.

That transition from their sometimes uncertain arms to big school was fraught with much fear, but not as much as I'd normally indulge in. Because he was better equipped on most fronts than I'd dared to dream.

And of course, I had my very first IEP papers in hand and the reassurance he was going to *the* best elementary school for balancing classroom inclusion and needed assistance. As well as a coveted appointment long in the making with someone named Dr. Kerschen, known to spot an autistic child in short order.

We bumped along with a very sensible, kind teacher and a general diagnosis of developmental delay until halfway into his kindergarten year. Then, at long last, we had our visit with the fabulous Dr. Kerschen who asked questions with a smile in her voice, let Elijah poke in all the drawers to her desk, and provided quite a sizable pile of both books and Megablocks to see the appointment through.

It wasn't long before she confirmed what we all had come to know, and that as much by watching him at play as through anything his teachers and I had filled in the bubbles on. Elijah was on the spectrum.

However, he still didn't fit the pigeonhole neatly. (In fact, whatever pigeonholes there are in life, he'll just walk away from and go invent his own, most likely.) So the official diagnosis was PDD-NOS (pervasive development disorder, not otherwise specified)—a fancy way of saying, yeah, he fits, but we don't know where.

But it's funny...I wasn't really all that frightened that day. Maybe because I was growing a little more used to visits and people poking in our heads with all those questions, or maybe because real answers were at last knitting together into something recognizable, but I attribute much to God using the dear lady's warmth and humor, her total love and embracing of kids like my Elijah to spill over into my brain and remind me that I *do* have allies in this world. My *kids* have allies in this world. There are those who do see worth in them and are interested not just in teaching them but in being taught by them.

This, to her, was not devastation, just difference, and that made all the difference to me.

I left that office still tired, honestly, but with new resolve to see to it Elijah had all he would ever need to succeed. And that others would see him for the grand person I always knew he was.

* * *

Now, if this was all I was facing in these years, it might seem a little overwhelming, but perhaps doable, you might say? Ah, but that was hardly all that occupied that time. Let us rewind a bit...

As soon as Elijah was first settled with therapists during his months at daycare, Timothy's teachers, two very wise and experienced ladies, approached me on the subject of testing him, purposely waiting until they thought I'd caught my breath.

Reassuring me that they both found him very verbal and bright at a little over two and a half, they raised concerns about his motor skills. Though I can say I had my moments of wondering on his part, the poor little guy had had to go so quickly from baby to being in the middle, I hadn't had the luxury to even worry on the same level as I had with Elijah. After all, he had tested out early from occupational therapy as a baby, and he was certainly chattier than his big brother at that age. But when they spoke of his struggles with his hands, I nodded my head in agreement, remembering my own fumbling from an early age and making the decision it would be better to intervene now than later.

So I again found myself in a flurry of paperwork, shaking hands and talking with numerous people who had conducted their tests, kind people who quickly assessed him as certainly *not* autistic. (Big breath exhaled right there, I must admit. I adore my autistic wonders with all my might, but I wasn't going to skimp on gratitude to God for the idea of at least one going through life without that particular struggle.)

Timothy was deemed very bright and interactive and extremely eager to please but with a body that wouldn't always cooperate with what he knew in his head how to do. While children on the spectrum tend to have struggles with their motor skills, Timothy's seemed to be a different breed of struggle, perhaps related to our family history of unofficially diagnosed joint conditions, myself included.

My initial thought was that genes can be cruel. Another awkward generation in a long line of klutzes. I wasn't terribly proud of such a thought, but there it was.

The recommendation was more occupational therapy and physical therapy as well. I just prayed for any kind of progress, feeling the weight of—at the time—not one but two kids in need of extra help. But what a gift God bestowed!

Watching Timothy work was amazing. Never did a child so young work so hard to succeed. By the time he was ready for kindergarten, he had exceeded expectations by far and tested out of therapy for the second time. (Today, there are a few residual struggles with opening things, lacing, handwriting, and the like, but those mountains are crumbling for him by the day.)

Well, you might be thinking, yes, two kids in therapy could be a bit harder than one... But we're not done yet... There's still baby Sarah. (She was christened thus by big brothers and remained so till she was three.)

Sarah was one of those plump, placid babies who entertained herself well from the start, typically with songs and stuffed animals. She was singing almost before she was talking. In lots of ways, this was a huge relief to a single, scrambling mama. Remember? I called her my consolation prize, a parting gift to get me through hard, lonely times.

I was loathe to leave her for the world of work, but so it had to be. In Grandma's loving arms, I left her to radiate joy wherever they went as well as learn the fun of silly games, books, and good old black and white sitcoms. (Her favorite for a long time was *The Munsters*. She could say *darn! darn!darn!* and flail her legs with the best of them.) She was nearly a year old when I began teaching, and she had yet to take those momentous first steps, but I wasn't worried. Elijah was almost thirteen months before he had taken his, and Timbo was about eleven months when he decided to chase after his brother unassisted on two feet, so no biggie. There was a wide range of normal on this, right?

17

Well, in the midst of everything I have already related, as the months ticked by, Sarah would occasionally pull up to furniture but wouldn't let go, and she still much preferred crawling to any other means of mobility.

"You probably carry her too much," came the snide remarks.

"Ummm...nooo. Just when it's a safety issue, as in across a crowded parking lot."

Some would shake their heads, unbelieving, and others would simply say, "Oh," and move on. Still others would say, "Well, it'll happen soon, and then you'll wonder why you wanted her to in the first place."

Very few offered any helpful answers, except for dear church members who offered prayer, joining with my own fervent ones. There was birthed in me an urgency to not leave this time around to chance. I was going to fight back for my kids in a bolder way, as prescribed by God. In addition, the previous experiences I now had under my belt with my boys would be fuel to spur me on with my only daughter.

In the meantime, the doctor had suggested if she wasn't walking by eighteen months, it was time to do what was called Screen for Success, a free comprehensive testing day to see where she was in various skills and perhaps get a clue as to where to go next. I was praying the whole time it wouldn't be necessary, but eighteen months came with nary a step, so I gulped, asked for yet more time off, and had my mom drive me to the church where it was held. (I don't drive. Short explanation: God is very capable, but some fears fall slowly. Manning a vehicle is my slow-falling one.)

She was sick as a dog, I recall, having caught some nasty bug that had laid me up the week before, but still she soldiered on and went, knowing it was the best opportunity to get help for months to come. Good ol' Mom, my right arm in so many adventures. Our childhood relationship of pain had morphed into a sort of Lucy and Ethel bond (without *too* many schemes and screw-ups).

Another very kind group of people put my little princess through her paces, watching her walk while holding my hands, testing hearing, sight, fine motor skills, speech. From there, it was deemed the process should begin to see what sort of therapies she'd benefit from.

There were visits to my parents' home and lists compiled of how many words she knew—roughly fifty at that time and deemed okay by their standards as long she continued to add vocabulary. Occupational therapy was, at the present, seen as unnecessary, but physical therapy was needed to get her on her feet and walking unassisted.

For the first time, I felt oddly at a distance from one of my kids' therapies—longing to see her walk and continuing to pray but not able to be as hands-on because of my work.

There was no way for Sarah to attend daycare with me. I taught her age group, and the policy at the time was that no parents were to teach their own kiddos.

I know my mom did what she could physically, limited as she was by her joints, and I tried to squeeze in the moments I could while still keeping our little world afloat. But for the first time in all my experiences with therapists, someone dropped the ball.

Visits suddenly stopped, vague answers were given, and frustration grew. Then, suddenly, in the middle of it all, at approximately twenty months, Sarah chose all by her little self to pick up and take her first wobbly steps.

Rightly or wrongly, busy and stressed as I was, I took it as my sign to let go of my worry, and I didn't pursue the matter further. It took time, but perhaps one child wouldn't struggle any further? Please, Lord?

But as time went on, Sarah continued to wobble, and not only that, her speech seemed in a holding pattern—not necessarily diminishing but not really flourishing. She also had some emotional sensitivities that seemed "normal toddler stuff" to the untrained eye, but—between my boys and my students, I now knew a little better what I should be seeing—I couldn't hide too long this time.

Sarah was still in need of help and, certainly, of further testing. When she reached two and a half, she was old enough to be a part of the next classroom over from mine, and she was soon added to the rolls. Between the three children, the paperwork that'd felt like flurries was now becoming a snowstorm as I cimbed on to ride the roller coaster once more.

It was with a tired but knowing manner I approached the matter this time. With chuckles about how I had enough copies of parental rights to wallpaper my apartment, we went through the various avenues of testing gross and fine motor skills, hearing (with screeches of protest when the nice people tried to invade her ears, something she dreads to this day), vision (using pictures instead of letters...she definitely recognized birthday cakes every time), and so on.

This time was not quite so scary as Elijah as I quickly saw the writing on the wall, and person after person was quicker to acknowledge the possibility of autism since older brother had a diagnosis. Before long, the recommendations were made, and as it turned out, their thoughts leaned in a different direction than they had with Elijah.

There was an elementary school down the street from my work where she could attend pre-k and receive all her services to boot. She could even qualify for a special bus to come pick her up from daycare. They absolutely loved her spirit and enthusiasm for life, which was so nice to hear, as she had had about as much struggle to be understood as Elijah had had in the daycare.

I went through yet another period of frustration at this point on that matter. I kept wondering where the knowledge they had learned in dealing with Elijah had gone. They seemed to be forgetting each child—even those on the spectrum—can be so different. So even with the trepidation of sending my only girl away for half the day, I was also a little relieved that she would be among those who were more educated in dealing with children like her.

After a bumpy start dealing with potty-training issues (By the way, did you know many autistic children have difficulty grasping the concept of potty training? No one told me till I had already done it!), Sarah settled beautifully into her routine.

Was every day perfect? No, but whose is?

The great part was her loving teachers who patiently coaxed growth out of her, all while delighting in her songs, her dances, and her joy. When she graduated and prepared for kindergarten at the school her brothers were in, there was much progress in her speech, her knowledge, and her motor skills. There were things yet to be worked on, as always with any child, but the nurture from those ladies had caused her to blossom. There were many tears and hugs and thanks going around graduation day. I will never forget those great people. Hopefully, they will read this and know their impact.

Actually, as I recall, it was there that one teacher made a profound statement during a conference that I have carried in my heart to this day. She herself was a mother to a then college-aged boy diagnosed with Asperger's Syndrome. (Some say this is part of the autism spectrum, some say it is not. I don't know where it currently sits, but suffice it to say, she could relate to me.)

In the course of chatting about our respective kiddos, she said, "Why does everyone always want to fix our kids? There's nothing wrong with them. They just think differently."

Yes! my spirit cried. *Thank you!* I can't say I never had frustrating days after that, but those words resonated with me again and again over the years, just as the lovely Dr. Kerschen did, who was again her warm, wonderful self when I brought Sarah in for her official diagnosis. Never did autism come across as something tragic when the word came from her. Rather, we laughed at Sarah's who-cares-what-you-think-I'm-gonna-sing-anyway attitude, just as we had laughed at Elijah's voracious curiosity just a few years ago.

Funny how pain falls away when you simply experience the joy that is your children. However God made them.

And so, in a manner of speaking, we had arrived. Ducks in a cockeyed sort of row.

No longer chasing diagnoses, but having them in hand for the chases that followed.

Chapter Three
Trucking Along,
Sometimes Singing a Song

With diagnosis times two in hand, you'd think life would become a little more settled. And, in a way, I suppose it did. We trucked along one year to the next, one IEP to another.

Typically, those meetings would be a big table of teachers, therapists, a pile of papers, and little old me, shy and nervous as a student myself. The first couple of years, invitations to the kids' dad were extended as well, but as with a lot of my life in those days, those texts and calls were forgotten.

So I found myself solitary, sometimes lonely, but not for long. Because in relating stories about my kiddos, laughter always tended—and still tends—to follow. I was blessed to be surrounded by such determined, caring, largely unflappable people. They knew, whether it was because of Elijah or Sarah's IEP or conference, to pencil in time to chat.

And even when the news wasn't as rosy—Elijah was still struggling with that argumentative nature, or Sarah was having a galloping case of the "I can'ts" in math or physical therapy—we nevertheless found much to laugh and marvel about, be it their unexpected brilliance in reading, baffling memory for things long forgotten by us adults, or their unparalleled enthusiasm for life demonstrated in songs in the hall or amazingly intricate origami.

And even though these meetings were never, obviously, about Timbo, conversation always arose about him as well—what a smart kid, what a devoted brother, older than his years (things I knew in my heart but delighted to hear nonetheless, especially because he was not only in the middle but was sandwiched by special needs, something I was ever conscious he not be eclipsed by).

Elijah's second-grade year brought about the next little jolt in our lives. He had skipped along through kindergarten and first grade with only a few bumps but had pretty much understood the information presented. It was, by and large, rote skills. Elijah understood rote skills. They were concrete. There were very few choices, very few steps.

Don't get me wrong. He is—and always has been—a creative, think-outside-the-box individual, but he is also a let-me-have-few-choices and don't-ask-me-to-pull-an-answer-from-thin-air kind of fellow when it comes to schoolwork and what he perceives as high-pressure situations—this could be anything from choosing between favorite meals to which video to pick out at the library. No biggie most times to you and me, but areas fraught with panic for him. Limits are his friend.

So second-grade social studies and essay questions began to get him down. Science, despite his passion for experiments and inventions, started tripping him up with abstract concepts out of his realm of interest. Math began to expand beyond that basic information, and he wound up somewhat lost, especially as expectations arose. "I don't know" became his go-to phrase on many of his papers. The natural tendency toward fidgets and inattentiveness that he has always possessed became more pronounced, more troublesome. Everyone still agreed he was so very sweet and personable in his way, particularly with adults, but for the first time, medication was recommended to hopefully help increase his focus.

Now, it couldn't be mandated—schools had no protocol to do so. I wasn't in love with the idea. To me, introducing medication to produce a more attentive student seemed to be, in a way, asking him to become a different child. But I highly respected the opinions of the ladies the suggestion was coming from. I looked at his floundering grades, then at his earnest but clearly stressed teachers, and agreed to check into the possibility.

So back I went to the wisest person I knew on this matter, Dr. Kerschen. We discussed every angle, every possibility, and came up with Adderall XR-to be taken every morning before school—that way it would be in his system throughout the entire day, the critical time for his attention to remain focused. After all, I was less concerned about the hours when *I* had him. Sure, I had to repeat myself a lot, but I was used to that. To me, that became my whole philosophy of dealing with autistic children—be patient and be prepared to repeat the message...many, many, many times.

At first, there was little noticeable change, but as enough medication was introduced to his system, we saw both the positives and the drawbacks. He was more in tune with the teachers during the school day, just as we'd hoped. But he was also less lively, less unfettered, more wakeful in the night, and more prone to emotional outbursts at home. He began to take a small dose of Adderall in the afternoon to ease his emotions, and this was the beginning of the end of my monkey boy and the ushering in of a somewhat better, quieter, but certainly more sober student. It was bittersweet. His grades saw an improvement about the same time shyness began to overtake him concerning things like music programs and special events at school. Every child faces such things in the maturing process, but it was almost as if the meds accelerated this.

Not that we haven't had our ups and downs still with attention and grades and so on, and not that he hasn't brought me countless smiles since, but there was something always less free than the boy who notoriously outsang the whole class singing "Gloria" in first grade. But then, I think every parent faces this point, don't they?

Sarah has fared better in this regard. While she undoubtedly has had her daydreaminess, her spontaneous bursting into song, and even the occasional alarming tendency to roam, she seems better equipped to sit and learn—and, in fact, even when she doesn't seem to be learning, she will astound us with the fact that she is. As far back as daycare, one of her teachers found she could shout out answers in circle time much better if she was allowed to sit in the library area and read while doing so. She was also known to do two puzzles at once in those days. I think this, too, speaks to how the autistic mind works, or at least some of them. Elijah shares this ability to an extent, but he typically has much preferred hand manipulation, his latest being doing origami while he listens. At any rate, the word *medication* has never fallen from the lips of any of *her* teachers yet, and hopefully never will. I don't think I could bear losing one ounce of her sunshine, and luckily, so far, neither could anyone who has worked with her. In a way, though, the disparate lack of tolerance there is between boys' and girls' behavior is maddening. There is more room for "daydreaminess" than "wiggles" in our schools today, and diminishing recess time sure doesn't help! (Oops. Soapbox. Don't trip over it!)

Okay. Back to the positive side…Elijah's third-grade year saw another change from the norm. For the first time ever, he had a male teacher, thanks to some excellent advice to request him for Elijah. This man was a fine example of a Christian as well as being well-versed in special needs, and thanks to his encouragement, Elijah experienced great academic strides, not to mention someone to connect with in his passion for superheroes at that time! I still recall how Spiderman, the major focus of his little mind, parlayed into a study of spiders in general and brought about one of the biggest triumphs Elijah had experienced to date—a well-written, detailed essay on black widows, complete with a truly awesome art project of a pipe cleaner spider complete with web. He was so proud of that project that it hung in his room for years to come, and it was with much sorrow (on mommy's part) that it was finally sacrificed as he made the decision he'd outgrown it. I still regret that one didn't get tucked in my humongous file cabinet of keepsakes, but there was no way of cramming it in there without damaging it!

I am an unabashed admirer of my children's efforts. I think most mamas are, but mamas of special needs children are even more so because every effort is so precious, another piece in the timeline of their learning. I can pull out an old paper from years before and relive the victory as well as marvel over how far they've come. It's also great when we've had a particularly down day, an unexpected setback, or an arduous tussle. It serves to remind me all they are capable of through Him who gives us strength.

Even now, I have to smile to myself at the way the Lord directs what I write about and when. We are at the beginnings of a new school year as I write this and grappling with a few less than stellar grades as the material takes the next step up for them. I have had some less than patient moments in my day, and honestly, in recent days, even as I preach to the masses more patience! More tolerance! (See? Even we moms of special needs who are so often told to feel "special" for being chosen by God to parent such kiddos are capable of appalling hypocrisy and lack of hope. Throws the saint theory right out the window, huh?)

Anyway, back to third grade... That was a happy year for Elijah, full of bright moments, though my favorite was a brief breakthrough in that wall concerning music that was going up.

It was the spring concert, and though I'd encouraged him to have fun with it, I'd about reconciled myself to watching him become stiff and uncomfortable and either barely moving his lips or not moving them at all—when I wasn't desperately trying to shush preschooler Sarah from singing over everybody, that is! And mostly, I was right until the class got to the old spiritual that goes "All night, all day, angels watching over me, my Lord."

I believe I had been fussing with Sarah just before, Timothy was in his usual "help Mom" mode, trying to coax little sis to sit by him in his cheeriest tone, and Mom was trying to help me with the both of them. But in spite of all that, the minute the music started, I looked up to pick Elijah out of the group. It was more to get it over with than anything, as I was expecting abject misery.

I was floored instead to find the most beautiful, peaceful expression on his face as he sang out, eyes closed, hands folded against his cheek. It was as though all faded from my sight but him, and he was the only child there. I think he felt it, too, though these days, whether he remembers depends on when you ask.

Even Sarah was quiet then, a miracle in and of itself. I knew he was talking to the God we were trying to teach him to understand, and I knew that he already *did* understand, more than any of us gave him credit for.

Still, it was a long time till I heard him sing like that again, and that has only been in recent times (when I am sneaky enough to catch him) as he discovered an area he could connect with: parody singers, particularly the Christian group Apologetix.

Now if I wanted to hear music, Sarah would—and will always—oblige, complete with sassy choreography, often accompanied by Timothy, my budding percussionist/electric guitar player, though we have learned she stays on key better on her own!

In the midst of Elijah's third grade year, she was getting set to graduate preschool—two separate schools and two separate ceremonies. She felt like a star. All the practicing songs and walking up to shake hands and receive diplomas…she took it all in stride.

I'm told it's odd for someone on the spectrum to so enjoy the limelight, but enjoy it she does…though admittedly, there are times even *she* has had enough—and that *did* happen at the daycare graduation.

By then, she had already done the one at her other school and had practiced for weeks, and she was tired. She lasted till the last song, and then, when they were supposed to go shaking their little booties down the aisleways, she ran straight for me.

It was with a twinge of sadness I wrapped her in my arms— she was almost there, after all, and she normally adores dancing—

but I quickly shook it off that night and told her how very proud I was of her. It doesn't do to dwell on your dreams of "perfect" experiences with your child, special needs or otherwise. (Pssst…it's because there aren't any!)

To use a somewhat hokey, mommy/baker's metaphor: Broken cookies taste just as sweet. Enjoy without loading yourself with the guilt. Goodness knows, I have had my share and have counseled my middle boy on the matter as I watched him develop with an alarming overabundance of the stuff.

As far back as the days "baby Sarah" was actually a baby, poor Timbo was developing lots of what I termed his "little old man" tendencies. I think much of it was being, as I referred to before, the one expected to be the "calm and mellow" center of an autism sandwich, coupled with losing a dad's daily presence before he was even walking.

Not all of this was bad, though, as by the time Elijah was in his third-grade year, Timothy was a very smart, sturdy, and eerily perceptive first grader, much beloved, extremely compassionate and helpful, loyal to his buddies, telling them all about Jesus's love for them. The hard part was when he actually dared to be human and make a mistake. He was—and still is—his own worst critic, be it a paper with more than a couple of missed questions, frustration with his hands not completing the task smoothly, or being corrected for minor infractions like talking a little too loud. And much like his mommy, he tries so hard to please that when he fails, he explodes on himself. And when others fail him, he tries so hard to tuck it away that, eventually, his mild-mannered ways give way to a verbal explosion on others.

I call this his "Hulk Smash" tendency. (It was no wonder he gravitated toward the big green guy when he was still in preschool. He's still a big favorite to this day.) I wish I could say I was always a great and patient example, but we have covered ad nauseum that I am no saint, right? :)

31

Over the years, he and I have stumbled together toward better ways and better esteem of ourselves. Usually, we can talk each other through those days we don't feel quite so up to the world we're living in or quite so up to our own expectations. Conversations with autistic children are so much fun most times, but it is often like trying to sort out words in two different dialects, so the ability to relate with Timothy, one to another, has been a solace for us both over the years. I often had my mom and dad in the midst as well in those days, but there were those times when they were busy, or I just wanted them to feel entitled to their own lives.

Those were the times, rightly or wrongly, I could confide in my middle son that I was feeling weary, and I knew he'd get it. I never wanted to treat him like a mini-adult, however. I tried hard to make sure he got equal attention and opportunity to whoop it up like the little boy he was. It just so happened that God graced him with what he'd need to survive this family, and it's often what I've needed, too. Amazing how He always knows, isn't it?

Chapter Four
Gotta Match?

As to myself and the depressions I had faced down in the midst of being a mom, I had gone from woebegone to angry to resigned. The separation period of my first marriage was prolonged, and as said before, I honestly prayed, holding out hope to the bitter end and beyond that somehow our fractured family would be restored. I extended the olive branch early on in a way many women would not in my case, but that isn't to say I'm a saint because, well, you know… :)

So I would say my angry period took a few good years to fully come into its own. I truly wrestled to maintain a Godly stance in all this, especially as I spent so much time meeting myself coming and going, and found fuel for the fire in my all-female workplace who had their understandably decided opinions about my situation.

Resentment grew that there was always so much to do, so many favors to ask my mom, yet no physical arms to lean on in the few quiet hours I had, no one to help shoulder the burdens as only a husband can. I know that could potentially raise the ire of single mothers everywhere who say, "Hey, I don't need a man!" I know it could also raise the ire of Christians who say to lean on the everlasting arms.

It's not to say I wasn't surviving pretty well or that I wasn't leaning on Him, but it's just that I had a problem. One I still possess to this day. I'm human!

My childhood was less than rosy (but if we're honest, whose was?). I had a rep as a weird, shy, goody-goody in school, no grand nor lucrative career, and now, I was watching my ex-husband go on with three more children, remarriage, and life. And yes, I resented how this pulled him away from our three— emotionally and financially. I resented how many times they expected to see him but were offered flimsy reasons why they couldn't and how I finally had to stop telling the kids about visits altogether until they materialized. I resented how I never had enough money to save.

Yes, there was a bitter root-seeking to take hold, and though many would call it justified, it wasn't pretty, and I didn't want it there. There was much time spent asking God to help me sort out my feelings, to pluck this root from my damaged heart.

Tears fell at a rapid rate so many days. It was a heavier burden for change than I'd known heretofore. But what change? And how to bring it about?

Then one day, I felt as though I had awakened from a long sleep. Something inside was telling me to let go. And I did. Of lots of things.

Of hopes and dreams I had erected for myself and my family.

Of the foolish hope and prideful, pious stance I held that somehow, someday, my ex-husband would wake up and return and of the belief that I was noble for praying for that for so long, of even the *desire* for him to return, but especially of the anger I had been unable to keep stuffing down so deep.

And it was then that I realized the romantic love had long since faded, and I was only punishing myself and my children by hanging on.

It was a freeing moment, and I wish I could say I remained cautious and prayerful after, but it doesn't take long for the devil to find a new crack to sneak through. Mine was found in, of all things, the accusation that I obviously wasn't that good at hearing from God (though I realize now it was the Holy Spirit's voice that had told me to let go) and therefore ought to just do things my own way. *Always a mistake!*

My own way consisted of signing up (with trembling hands) with Match.com, seeing as I didn't have time to meet anyone in my come-and-go existence.

My first write-up was honest but full of baggage and Christianese, so not much was garnered at first. For a time, I did more searching for profiles than receiving responses. The first one I truly tangled with was funny and odd…and a church-goer-turned-atheist. That should've made me run screaming, but loneliness overtook sense, and I spent the next few months attempting to "convert" him, instead finding myself sinking into darkness quite rapidly as our collective insecurities dragged both of us down.

When that situation had played itself out, I rewrote my profile with a more jaded air, attracting one poor situation after the next, trying to affect a stony disattachment, yet longing deep down to find someone who believed as I did, who was interested in the kids and their needs. (I had adopted what I felt was a good policy of not introducing the kids to anyone so they wouldn't get attached, but honestly, no one really offered anyway.)

My mom was incredibly patient and always there to lend advice and babysitting. She was rightly worried about this rabble I was meeting up with, but of course, in my latent rebellion, I took her up on the babysitting far more than the advice.

And then, my grandparents passed—first my grandmother from prolonged illness following a stroke and then my grandfather two weeks after from undiagnosed COPD and, I believe, a sense he no longer had to hold on now that his wife was gone.

Theirs was a long, tumultuous, but ultimately redemptive relationship as I saw it (though some family may not be able to see it that way). I ended up in a brief but very real emotional tailspin as I realized none of the men I went out with had the salt to stick by me as PaPa and Granny had to each other, or even the salt to be any measure of comfort in this loss.

Here I was, surrounded by people but still so alone. It was then I briefly decided I was about ready to chuck it all. Now, to be frank, it was not my first brush with suicidal thoughts. I had battled those since middle school. It's never ever a good thing—nor a right thing—but truly, there is no more terrible feeling than, as a mother, facing the desire to end your own life. There is the guilt that you aren't enough to your kids in your current state of living and the guilt of even considering the possibility of leaving them. It is a dangerous precipice to stand on and one I don't wish on anybody.

A lot of people preached a lot of things to me in this time, but honestly, it was, once again, when I looked into three pairs of beautiful brown eyes that adored me and needed me that I really realized I couldn't leave them behind. Thus, with much prayer and a shaky but determined hand honestly extended for help beyond my own four walls to that dreaded but necessary therapist, suicide was at long last laid to rest in me.

After all, there was so much yet to discover together in our own unique, stumbly-bumbly way. And who better to trip along with my beauties than the main constant God had thus far graced them with? There had to be purpose in it all.

And shortly thereafter, I was to find a new aspect to it all.

Another large piece of my solution had been to cool my jets and chuck Match.com instead of chucking me. First, though, I couldn't resist doing one more perusal just for kicks…

And then, as can only happen with a God who delights in serendipity and eleventh-hour surprises, I saw *him*. **My Joe.**

Match had never paired us, he had never seen my profile, and in all my searches, I had never seen his up to this point. He had twinkling blue eyes and an ornery but not obnoxious smile. His words weren't many, nor were they necessarily poetic. He spoke a great deal on the simple life and his desire to find someone who was similarly inclined. Something about that resonated with me.

After so much complication in my life, simplicity sounded like a feathery pillow to rest on after scraping by for so long on hard, cold gravel.

I had my serious doubts he'd reply—the nice ones rarely did—but I felt so compelled to tell him how much I liked what he had to say that, before I could chicken out, I wrote him as honest an e-mail as I could stand. I was even transparent enough to say I doubted he'd reply, a big boo-boo in all those "project self-confidence" books.

And…when the reply didn't come fairly quickly, I figured he had checked out my profile and dismissed me as I had feared. I went around feeling oddly vindicated, though definitely not happy to be so. (Funny, though, that I had all but forgotten my plan to drop out of Match in this process of sit back—ok, perch anxiously—on my chair and wait.)

Lo and behold, just as I had shrugged it all off as yet another washout, a couple of days later, I got a beep on my phone. Joeu977 has sent you mail! I couldn't help myself. I eagerly got on the site and retrieved it, preparing all the while for a "thanks, but no thanks," as the nicest guys usually sent those, but I opened it to find a very friendly reply that let me know two things right off the bat.

His top priorities? God and family. I admit it. My jaw dropped. I quickly wrote back an unabashed "Me, too!!!"

From there, we conversed pretty well, exchanging phone numbers for ease of conversation because he drove a truck in those days. (Now I knew why the reply took a couple of days! *See, Ms. Cynic?* God seemed to delight in saying.)

His estimation continued to rise in my eyes. He didn't hold back about himself, but he didn't blabber on trying to impress. (I was sooo happy, for example, that he didn't promise to take me out dancing. We both had two left feet and were unashamed to say so!) But more than anything, when he began to ask about the kids, and all—I repeat, ALL—the ins and outs of autism and how that affected them, my heart rose higher still as I finally had someone who wanted to hear my stories of triumph and defeat.

And finally, we decided we had had enough of the phone, and it was time to meet in person. I was nervous about this step because disappointment had inevitably followed every other time. But he went and made himself that much more a hero in my eyes when he asked me to bring the kids and even offered to take them to their version of the grandest place on earth: McDonald's (or "Old McDonald's" as the kids used to call it, often singing its virtues in their made-up song, "Old McDonald's had a cheeseburger, yummy, yummy, yum!").

Needless to say, they were over the moon to be accompanying me on one those mysterious dates they had always heard Grandma and me discussing. After all, they'd never gone before!

There just happened to be one of those red-clown palaces catty-corner to our apartment complex, so we agreed to meet for dinner, my mom playing chauffeur as per usual—and not-so-secret inspector. She was thrilled to be able to check one of these guys out, as she had only met one other, and that one by taking him by surprise at his workplace.

Oh, I remember well the fizzy feeling of anticipation knotting in my stomach as we pulled into the lot, like butterflies flapping their wings and knitting their antennae together in a sea of shaken Sprite.

I spotted him pretty quickly—long and lean, posed against his old Ford truck. He wore his trademark ball cap and a boyish smile under his whiskers. A little bit scruffy and a tad bit wolfish, but not intimidatingly so.

The kids whispered excitedly to each other in the back seat, craning their necks for a better view as he loped on those tall man's legs across the lot to my mom's car.

My troop piled out, and he actually did the sweet, increasingly rare thing and went to shake my mom's hand. She told me later he was the first man I had dated she felt no fear about, and I know that was a part of why.

Another reason was the moment he walked up and spoke, she saw the uncanny resemblance to my recently deceased PaPa! (By the way, anybody who thinks things happen by chance doesn't know much about God's humor, His delight in comforting his children, or His expert timing! Right down to crawdad-eating, loving jalapenos, and a fascination with fixing things, God brought back so many things that reminded us of PaPa through my Joe.)

And then, we were all inside the French-fry warmth and colorful cacophony of our favorite spot. He handled the complicated orders—noooo pickles for Elijah Bear, chicken nuggets and loooots of ketchup for the princess, absolutely positively no ketchup for Timbo, and plain burger for the weird mommy—with aplomb.

Not to mention the ease with which he handled following the hour-long "Muscle Man" story Elijah insisted on sharing. It was Elijah's personal amalgamation of Spiderman, Hulk, Iron Man, and Spongebob Squarepants, and his fasciniation lasted for an intense duration of two and a half years, a near record for Elijah as his likes tend to last only one year. (*Blue's Clues* was the only real exception. He would never say so outright at the ripe old age of thirteen, but there is still a fondness there as for a first love.)

The thing about Muscle Man was he was much more often told than ever written down or drawn (even though Elijah is quite talented in both regards). The other thing was the plots were nearly entirely lifted from *Spongebob* episodes with only names and a few details changed. Elijah was fairly animated but difficult to pause. I know it had to have been tough to listen that entire dinner, but listen Joe did, turning to me occasionally with dimpled smiles and a whispered comment or two. After all, he was supposed to be dating me, too, right? :)

Of course, the kids figured they had as much right to monopolize our new friend as I did. Even Timothy was more animated than usual, putting his little bits of flavor into Elijah's story as "Dr. Green." (Gee, who is *that* supposed to be like? I *do* love the fact Elijah accommodated his brother's love of the Hulk there. Some wrongly assume autistics are almost incapable of thinking about others, but while we have had our times of needing to teach social appropriateness, my kiddos seem to possess enough compassion to shame most adults.)

But the crowning moment of the night was Sarah. This is the part of the "how we met" story we fight (good-naturedly, of course) to get to tell. My little princess had been sitting across from us all evening, happily munching her ketchup-drowned nuggets and guzzling chocolate milk, not saying much but occasionally peeping at the funny whiskered man next to me.

When she was done, she got it in her head to get up and squeeze between us. *Uh-oh,* I thought, as she caused him to have to scooch over in the booth. *What is she up to?* Next thing I knew, she was slipping one arm around each of us, glancing from one to the other with a solemn expression.

Then she stated matter-of-factly, "You two on a date. You two gonna get married." She broke into a radiant smile about the time I turned as red as Ronald McDonald's hair. I didn't dare look at Joe, but I heard him half-cough, half-chuckle and figured he was about as red.

I think I mumbled something about her tendency for bluntness and her overexposure to Cinderella stuff. We recovered, though, and he didn't go running or shutting down. He even requested a picture of us for his phone. Elijah took it for us.

Looking back on it, we both looked petrified, yet we were at the beginning of an amazing journey. And as he offered to walk us home that crisp November night, with Sarah begging to ride piggyback on his shoulders (which she would never do with someone she couldn't trust) and the boys tagging along close to his side, me leading the way but glancing back often to see all this and marvel at it, I halfway dared to think that yes, it might be possible. Maybe, just maybe, God had indeed looked down, saw the mess I was creating, and plucked me out to put me on the path he had meant for me all along...

Chapter Five
Shotgun Wedding
Minus the Shotgun

And with those words fresh in my head, you'd think I'd finally just surrender to God's plan for me, straighten up and fly right and so forth, but again, um, *human*. No saints here.

I dearly wish I could say that this is one situation I approached with a clear head, but alas, I was *so* frightened. The possibility of someone who could actually fully embrace me and my ragtag band was so fantastic I could hardly dare to believe it. In my experience, such promises proved to be mere illusions. So it was with equal parts romantic abandon and protective instincts that I approached this change in our existence.

One moment, I'd find myself recklessly running into Joe's arms, professing my love, allowing temptation to take over. The next, I would be swimming in regret, running in fear before *he* could... And yet, he never did, and he never let me run too far, either, to my extreme befuddlement.

I think I equally befuddled him. He'd had a long, hard life. Adoption following abuse as a young boy, a mixed-up youth filled with trying and failing to squeeze in, and then turning to drugs, alcohol, and theft that eventually saw him a vulnerable seventeen-year-old at Lansing prison.

And then, God got a hold of him, and he never looked back.

He told me all this early on, expecting a swift kick out the door as so many had done despite time and powerful testimony. But my first thought was, who was I to judge a past?

I, who had survived abuse, abandonment, and a very lonely, struggly, mixed-up time of it myself? It wasn't and still isn't always easy or smooth to overcome, but really, as I think on it even today, who better to help each other overcome than two people who have been in similar places?

My prison walls may've been different, but they were there in my life as much as his were in those nine years of imprisonment. And for both of us, they are yet a part of who we are today.

And besides, there was so much joy flowing in the midst of it all. Bonds were forming, and the kids were truly thrilled with the novelty of a man around the house and seeing their mommy in a better humor than they had seen in so long, although Elijah could've done without the "lovey-dovey."

I still laugh when I remember the first time he saw us kiss. His nine-year-old brain couldn't fathom that it could be pleasurable. Even though his favorite movie at the time was Spiderman, he'd run from the room when Peter Parker and MJ lip-locked. He had actually said, "Ewww," stopping us mid-kiss. We broke out in embarrassed giggles, unable to continue at that point.

We even spent Thanksgiving together, a small, casual affair as only my folks could have—sitting around their apartment with plates of turkey and stuffing, and the kids having their own individual favorites and watching cartoons and classic TV. I knew Joe came from a big family that probably celebrated on a far grander scale, so I did wonder how he'd feel about our little celebration, but he rolled along with us in great spirits, eating with gusto and making us all laugh as only he could—and still can. It was as if he'd always been there...and what a comfort on our first holiday after my grandparents' passing.

We had both of us already secretly discussed marriage— frightening in the fact we had only known one another for weeks, and equally frightening in that it felt so right. I treasured all this in my heart, not quite ready to firmly plan things, but my giddiness was certainly evident to all from kids to parents to coworkers. Looking back, I am fairly sure some were nauseous at our gooey state of being, but then, of course, there was also mixed in there the (finally!) feeling of relief from all who saw me go from lonely single mom to frustrated dater to this present happiness.

And then the moment of reckless abandon came home to roost. I was late—as in my bodily functions were late—and if there was one thing I never was, it was late for my monthly, errr, appointment. Except for the times I was expecting.

So the first step—after a swift and repentant collapse to my knees—was to scrape up as much courage as I possibly could in my shaky little expectant self and tell Joe.

Though the idea of marriage had already been tossed around more than once, I prepared myself for the strong possibility he might not stand by me, especially when I considered the relationship was still rather new to bear up under such a monkey wrench.

I don't remember just what words tumbled from my trembly lips, but I do recall my mouth felt like it was full of wallpaper paste, and my hands uncategorically refused stillness.

And then, I remember the wait. Expectant of an explosion followed summarily by so long, goodbye, see you in the funny papers.

Yet again, he surprised me with a measured calm and a sense of it's-happened-so-let's-go-with-it I'd had little experience with in my thirty-plus years of mass hysteria.

Though I know inwardly he was as stricken as I from guilt, shame, and fear, he never unloaded that on me and fully acknowledged our equal parts in this sin and the urgency to tend to the results. We made the trip together to get *the* test, came home, and took it. When the little pink plus sign showed up, it was truly no surprise but mere confirmation. We embraced, wept, and began to resign ourselves to the fact we were to be parents—for me, for the fourth time, and for him, the first—albeit through a highly imperfect set of circumstances.

And now, we had two families to face with this news. We were thirty-three and thirty-four, respectively, but such a daunting task nevertheless reduced us both to awkward children.

I naturally feared mass hysteria would make its unwelcome return on my end and on his. For me, at least, there was such a paralyzing notion of the utter unknown.

At that point, I had yet to even meet his parents. It'd been discussed, but though they were definitely thrilled with the fact he'd met someone, they'd had, well, a lot of experience with disappointments in their middle child's life, so we'd held off on that first meeting. Now, I feared all the more what they'd think of me.

I wasn't privy to the conversation that went down between the three of them, but suffice it to say, they were adamant Joe do right by me and take care of the life created. Honestly, looking back, it was a scary, scary time, but it warms my heart that they were concerned for my welfare from the get-go. I felt like the "hussy" that had lured their son, yet they were concerned for *me*.

With that hurdle cleared, I breathed a bit, yet there was still *my* family left. A whole different level of fear. Telling my parents anything, much less a "your squeaky-clean girl screwed up big time" thing, really did reduce me to the days I was in middle school bringing home a bad grade. We knew we could hold off a little while, and we were certainly waiting to tell the kids, so we decided to not (potentially) ruin Christmas. We'd hold back till New Year's to share our news.

The first Christmas went off without a hitch, other than the famous "wreck of our first real Christmas tree" by Joe's miniature lab Ricky, left alone in my apartment for the first—and last—time. He was a Houdini of the wire crate. Hence he ended up staying with me and the kiddos (who were so happy and giggly about having our first pet on premises) as a last resort. The cost for him to ride in Joe's truck was prohibitive. Unfortunately, the cost to my rented apartment also proved prohibitive.

When I called up Joe in his truck to describe my torn blinds and my new carpet of pine needles and broken ornaments, as well as dear Sarah's pronouncement of "bad dog, bad dog," I again fully expected to be sent on my way—after all, you don't come between a man and his dog. But God again graciously let me know this man was serious when his unhesitant instructions were to give Ricky away in order to relieve my stress.

All that aside, it was a lovely Christmas beyond anything I could imagine in my long, bleak winters without anyone to wrap an arm around me while watching twinkling reds and greens or participating in raucous present opening.

Joe was a big hero to the kids that year, fulfilling dreams of real walkie-talkies, science kits, and pretty princessy books and crayons as well as sharing in what we as a family always loved doing, whether it was favorite Christmas specials (Charlie Brown is the man) or looking at lights. And I had the pleasure of someone to give something to after all these years (a Bible cover I agonized over) and someone to give something to me—beyond the ornaments the kids labored on in school, precious as those are and will always be.

He'd already given lots of spontaneous things—my first being a beautiful sign that hangs proudly in our living room today bearing the words: Dream. Home is the Starting Place for Love and Dreams. Already I was filled with such a sense of warmth and security wrapped in the knowledge he wanted to extend such words to my too-often-hopeless soul.

But for Christmas, he decided I needed more than mere words on an old wooden plaque. I also needed a ring to seal this promise to stick around for the long haul.

Now, there is just something about being taken to pick out something like that. It's surreal. Someone wanted to spend all that hard-earned money on *me*. Someone wanted to let the world know he'd picked *me*. On purpose.

So...of course, I went single mom practical and talked him down in the price range he wanted to spend. I had to tell him over and over I was perfectly thrilled to have my simple intertwined hearts. (Still thrilled, by the way. Life's too short to spend on doo-dads when you can spend it on something lasting.)

So by then, I had an engagement ring, and we'd even discussed a March 17 wedding date. My folks were growing comfortable with the idea of an impending marriage, so much so that Dad even jokingly called us "Joseph and Mary" and, unbeknownst to him at the time, made us squirm with laughing comments of an "immaculate conception."

Still, we figured the groundwork was laid, and it was time we got it over with. The kids were on a rare visit to their biological father's, so we dug out my favorite board game, Scrabble, and trooped the forty steps from my apartment to my parents' to play a marathon session to ring in the new year, just the four of us.

Joe had promised to help me break the ice, and that he did. We had been making chit-chat as we laid down our words, making up stories to go along with them, having a great time, when he just happened to get the letters L-A-T-E. Seeing his opening, he laid them down and off-handedly mentioned someone in the room was "late."

Always perceptive, my mother understood first. My dad, ever sweet and naive, needed a little more help putting it all together. But when Mom had gotten it into his head, here's the amazing part...while I sat with bowed head, pink cheeks, and a boatload of shame welling up afresh, my mom and dad were nodding their heads rather peacefully.

Somehow, time and God's grace had done the ever-astounding job nothing else can. It helped them to remember they had been in a similar position some thirty-seven years before and extended the understanding they had missed out on as frightened teenagers.

That isn't to say it was their proudest moment as my parents, but what could've divided that day drew us even nearer than we'd been before, and the determination was made to pick up and go on with the help of God's ever-guiding hand.

And so wedding plans were underway—not because it was necessarily a "had to" situation. We have reiterated often we'd have married regardless of the results of the test that day. But we saw no reason to prolong things, either, as everyone from parents to kiddos were onboard, and, okay, also because few women *really* want to either be a parade float on their wedding day or tote a squalling newborn down the aisle. (Censure me if you will, but I am just stating my own thoughts on the matter!)

The March 17 wedding date had surfaced first as somewhat of a joke—Joe is a dear, sweet, forgetful man, so I couldn't resist teasing him about picking a memorable date. However, it quickly morphed into a serious idea, green theme and all.

The kids got right into the spirit of things, finding green clothes and decor, enthusiastically jumping on ideas of green punch (which wound up staining all our tongues emerald), truly awesome fuzzy green antenna (for them) and afro wigs (for Joe and I) so we could make a fun, goofy surprise entrance to the reception, and a cake decorated with green M&Ms in expert fashion by my talented mother-in-law, who quickly became a new ally for my kiddos.

Her innate understanding was mystifying at first until she introduced a new wrinkle that summed it all up to me—the man I was about to marry had no official diagnosis of high functioning autism, but all the traits were there in his growing up years! He himself never knew until she found out we were getting married.

I pondered for a bit how it must've felt to suddenly find this out, but two great things were born of this late reveal: one, we saw how not being pigeonholed freed him from being unfairly judged or held back, as society too often labels those who process differently, and two, we realized it was no wonder he could read the kids so well, especially Elijah, who shares so much of his adoptive father's traits from insatiable curiosity to nearly impenetrable stubbornness.

There may've been that rough period of finding himself, of course—something not to be wished on anyone—but in the end, he was shaped by it all.

And then, of course, here was yet another opportunity to marvel at how God attends to every detail in our lives, sewing up every stitch with love and grace and astounding care, knowing just what we need and when.

My love for Joe didn't diminish one iota but rather grew as I gained further insight into his amazing character and reveled in the proof that autism needn't stop anyone from succeeding as a human being.

In fact, it can *enhance* success by reminding us that the qualities of integrity and transparency we don't revere enough are often a large part of what makes people on the spectrum tick. My hope was buoyant at this point. Fear tried to mix in there as it can with us insecure, "burned" folks, but as the wedding day approached, it really melted away.

* * *

It had been kind of iffy weather in the last few days (typical Kansas), but March 17 was sunny and mostly mild with just a bit of wind blowing.

The wedding was beautiful and so full of the stuff of my family from Sarah (escorted by Timothy) as flower girl attempting to pick up the petals sprinkled down the aisle with an innocent exclamation of "Oh! You dropped some!" to Elijah's super solemn walk with the rings alongside his soon-to-be cousin to Dad concentrating heavily on not messing up the wedding march as he walked me down the aisle to Michael W. Smith's Agnus Dei.

The crowning moment came, however, when Joe's ring got stuck halfway on—his knuckle is an unusual size—and he tried to slip it on all through the titters that followed during the rest of the pastor's pronouncements. (He got it on in time for our kiss, and, truth be known, it's rarely ever come off aside from once or twice to clean it.)

Not that it was all laughs. We knew it was as significant an event in the kids' lives as in ours, so we wanted to be sure they got to participate in a very special way beyond the norm. We chose to do two things:

First, each of us had colored sand we poured into a large glass vase to symbolize the blending of our lives. Second, Joe made vows to them as inspired by the movie *Courageous*. (Watch it if you never have, but arm yourself with Kleenex! If you've seen it, you know what I mean.)

This was perhaps the most touching moment of all for me, watching the wonder on my children's faces as Joe, with tears pouring down his face, vowed to be the father God wanted him to be. It's sometimes hard to know how much my children absorb in such a pinnacle moment because emotion is such a maze for them to navigate at times, but I knew that day that they knew their new daddy's love for them. There was neither doubt nor confusion on their faces. Only awe.

Their young lives had changed in perhaps the biggest shift ever, even beyond their natural father's leaving or the diagnoses of autism. For this would set them on a road of challenges heretofore never faced as well as growth none of us could have ever anticipated.

Chapter Six
First Year Festivities and Fumbles

To say we had a honeymoon period would be somewhat true, but honestly, those of you out there with blended families and clamoring responsibilities know it takes a lot of balancing and stretching, a lot of muscle and know-how to make the wheels of your new family go.

Add to that moving to a new apartment, two special needs children and a third you don't want to feel forgotten, a daddy driving a truck the better part of the week, and a mommy with an ever-burgeoning pregnant belly still running/waddling after a class of toddlers at work, and the gymnastics get that much more advanced. To fit in time for sentiment, you must be very deliberate.

Frankly, we are *still* in the midst of that process, but we have been slowly mastering the art of a generous learning curve at the feet of a gracious heavenly Father who didn't give us the flunking grades we deserved but started us with a clean slate instead.

Setting up new digs was rather exciting, even in seemingly mundane ways. For the first time in years, I had a bedroom! There are many sacrifices made on a less-than-wealthy single mama's road sometimes. One of mine had been to sleep on a daybed in my living room for three years. (Not too shabby when it comes to watching TV and snacking in bed. Everything was conveniently located!)

Not to mention I now had a very capable pair of hands to help where I'd always struggled. Someone with whom to discuss school and kids and finances and the frustrations of teaching and trucking. Someone to accompany me to doctor appointments for my baby-to-be and me. Someone to share the couch with me at night and the row of chairs at church.

It was a season of utter exhilaration and a celebration of our God and His infinite goodness. I looked forward to every phone call while Joe was hard at work on the road, and my ears strained to hear his every homecoming.

I learned to make coffee and real dinners, and I slowly watched the kids' classic autistic and just plain picky food issues dissipate as Dad put his foot down.

Trying to give him room to contribute on such things was odd at times. I knew it was necessary to allow him to shape his approach, gain respect, and establish relationships. Yet a sort of contention began to eke through as the months wore on. Sometimes it felt like he was trying to change my babies overnight or discount what we had accomplished over the years. There were some harsh tones that caught us off-guard. Expectations that took us aback.

I soon found myself spouting off my thoughts in return and swooping in to defend my territory, and the first hints of a wall rose up.

Particularly, Elijah, being oldest and so eerily like Joe, both faced the ire and dished out a fair amount of it. Having entered his double-digit years and in need of guidance at about the same moment he most resented it, he found his voice and used it. Often.

And with a dad who had only just inherited the duties of three and one-in-the-making, the balance of power was rocked.

Elijah had rarely had to answer to a dad in his young life. Visits to his biological father were more about loosey-goosey fun than any attempts at molding. My own dad strived to instill some things as he could, God bless him, but being on the road himself much of the time made this difficult to achieve most days.

So…

For Elijah to suddenly be thrust into this new life of answering to a male figure on a regular basis was strange for him. At times, strangely comforting. But mostly, just strange.

Joe, for his part, was working with what he knew. His parents were lovely people who brooked no nonsense. So a lot of what I attributed to the typical behaviors of autistics were deemed things that could be eradicated.

To my dear husband's credit, he was correct in some assessments. It was wonderful to see them eat—and not just McNuggets and burgers—as well as to gain in areas of personal responsibility and physical prowess.

Bu in others? Well, the battles over some things became legendary in our household.

His patience in terms of forgetfulness, curiosity, and all those childhood foibles that needn't even be attached to an autism label was sometimes too short for my taste. His sternness over table manners and some other things I had chosen not to battle in my busy and often flat-out tired state for so many years. These things were significantly more important to Joe.

It was startling to see us through someone else's eyes. Startling…and a bit deflating.

At times, I think I just wanted him to relax more. After all, we had so little time while he was home. I sometimes became the distressed child I once was, just wanting all the raised voices to quiet, to feel acceptable despite faults, and to see peace reign in our lives as it had in the first bloom of our relationship.

We were newlyweds, after all. Shouldn't we *feel* more like that? Where was that rosy hue of elation that had once colored our little world?

I even began to question what I knew I ought not to question— but did anyway as a woman once abandoned. Was this more than he had initially signed up for? Had the promised product disappointed upon bringing it home? Would he grow displeased enough to leave? After all, he was on the road a lot anyway. Plenty of opportunity to keep on trucking right out of our lives. Isn't that what guys do when you are just too much luggage for the promised long haul?

Vows are vows after all, but with a self-proclaimed screw-up like me, weren't they always proved conditional?

It wasn't really that anything in *his* behavior, while at times a little quick-on-the-draw, a little on the overly charming side with females, would give me any concrete reason to question loyalty. It was just the place I went to—and continue to fight against going to—as one whose confidence in oneself was always precarious at best and, at worst, a shambles.

It wasn't to say we never had our happy times in those early days of formation. For every wounding, battling time, there were dozens of delightful days. Light and full of off-the-wall humor. Goofy, playful, down-to-earth family days that were so gorgeous I thought my heart might break from the sheer joy of it. The feeling—finally—that this was our new reality.

We were none of us walking this life alone. We had each other.

From the breathless beauty of looking on our baby boy-to-come with a husband who'd never gotten to see something of his own on an ultrasound to the humble sweet feeling of actually, finally getting a baby shower on the fourth child thanks to my loving mother-in-law, there were so many genuine smiles and happy tears.

And from the childlike fun of watching a new dad teach the kids how to properly mold a snowman to watching him become their video game hero, there was much we could find ourselves blending on even as there was much we struggled to come together in. Like a toddler finding his legs, we were slowly bending knees and testing our feet to find out how to stand.

And then...I got gestational diabetes, something I'd never encountered in three rather uneventful pregnancies prior to this. And I had to learn to go from a sugarholic, big-time bread-eater to blood-testing, carefully weighing portions, and embracing a more veggie sort of lifestyle.

I knew it was good for me and good for my baby, so as I did with many other things in my life, I just marched on and did it. Because I *had* to.

Yet while I blessedly remained diet-controlled and never had to inject a drop of insulin, I was definitely tired. More than tired. Weary would be a better word. I was thirty-four and no spring chicken as a few liked to remind me. I bristled at that thought when so many women do it all so well, it seemed, and were older than me! But the droopiness was swiftly evident enough that each day saw me dragging my feet more. My lesson plans, while still creative, became more daunting to write, and my students were not so much a source of sunshine as an obligation to consider.

My plan was to stay on until summer, giving me a couple of months with the older kids till baby boy made his entrance in August, but near April's end, I saw I just wasn't going to make it.

With that insecure quaver in my voice I just can't conceal well, I asked Joe about leaving sooner, partially fearing a scolding for not being stronger or thinking harder about the money. Yet again he showed love and tenderness as he told me to do what I needed. We'd be fine. I wasn't scrambling in the financial dark anymore. There was, in fact, someone to partner with me in keeping the checkbook alive now.

I knew this before, but sometimes the mentalities we train ourselves to live in take time to truly shed. I'd grown so used to the single mom shuffle I often forgot I wasn't in this alone anymore.

And so, feeling the release I needed to pick up my oil crayons and kiddie songs and move on, the chapter begun nearly six years before came to a close rather more suddenly than anticipated. It was bittersweet to shut the door on the place that had sheltered me in my green days, had grown me up in lots of ways, and had guided three of my children in some of their wobbliest moments, not to mention mine.

It hadn't always been perfect, to be sure, but it was honestly more than just a job by the time all was said and done. It had become a window into lives and people and circumstances my bruised existence had gleaned much from—more than I could've anticipated at the outset.

Yet there *was* a sizable measure of relief in walking away and leaving it behind before I collapsed or became anything more diminished to my dear students than I'd already seen myself becoming. They mattered far too much for me to let that happen.

There are days I look back fondly and miss it, but then I realize doors open and close many times in our lives. A big piece of our existence is transition.

Max, our beloved black dachshund-mini lab mix, came to us at this time to restore what Joe had sacrificed in losing Ricky. Max was and is a sweet companion and protector, a little abandoned soul in his own right. He was rescued from the shelter, which had, in turn, rescued him from a lonely country existence of stealing chickens and roaming without family. Needless to say, he tugged at something deep inside me that day, quietly approaching and hopefully sniffing us, cautiously wagging his tail, grateful for good petting and kind voices.

We went into the shelter for "just a look" that Sunday afternoon but found ourselves unable to leave without this orphaned soul so kindred to us. And he swiftly dug a path into our hearts—and gave me a refresher on taking care of a needy little one!

The kids certainly enjoyed *this* particular transition and were eager to pitch in with his care. It was good to watch their growth in this area, tenderness and a sense of duty emerging in my rapidly maturing brood.

And a few short months later, another needy one, another heart-expanding addition was ready to come...

Chapter Seven
Baby Has Left the Building— and Entered Our Hearts

David John, as we'd come to call him while still in the womb— honoring my uncle who departed this world far too tragically at age four and my grandfather who'd passed when I was three—was doing a funny sort of thing to me toward the winding down of that stereotypically long, hot summer.

Due date impending, he absolutely refused to right himself for his exit. The already ornery little guy was insistent on feet first no matter how often checked.

Painful procedures loomed to attempt physical persuasion in getting him to shift, ones that were apparently only shots in the dark as to success. The word C-section floated around as well.

The doctor advocated for the manual shifting thing, but I honestly was terrified of this unknown. I'm very sure many have done this without so much as a howdy-do, but, well, I am sort of a chicken.

C-section was my request, or rather, it was what I settled for since the little tyke was stubbornly set.

Being cut open was no fun at all, but at least it was a familiar pain. I could do the stitches again, I thought. Well, maybe.

The real challenge would be the stairs in our townhouse. Climbing with that constant burning tug on your tummy would probably not be doable for a while.

And honestly, the recovery would be longer, which kind of stinks for the wife of a trucker whose paycheck we'd need before I'd be up and bouncing.

My heart began to sink as I considered all this.

Yet sweet Joe told me not to worry. As always.

Mom and Dad naturally offered their assistance, too. Very much welcome, of course.

It'd be okay. It would. But I still found myself frightened despite all the reassurances. I did a lot of breathing in and out and a lot of crying, praying, and crying some more.

The Sunday before one last ultrasound, which was to be followed by the scheduled C-section, I was in church with all this weight heavy on my shoulders, striving to shake it off in praise. And failing miserably to achieve it on my two puffy feet. This song began that I had always found odd for church—even in that lively, untraditional place we were attending back then. Its lyrics said something about how God turns situations around, upside down, inside out. Something about feeling a shift. Words that resonated deep in my anxiety-ridden heart. Things I was longing for in a very literal way.

Almost automatically, my hand slid down to cradle my belly and the sweet little life therein. I was raised Charismatic, but frankly, I didn't and don't jump aboard every sign that comes down the pike. Parts of me resist, parts of me feel like too many jump aboard too many bandwagons. (Ah, but that's truly a different story for a different time.) That said, this felt like another moment God was tugging gently at me, smiling down with a secret on His lips.

"Take it, daughter," I heard His tender urging. "It's for you."

So I sang out even though it wasn't my favorite song. And I danced as best as a woman with a watermelon in her dress could.

Later, I confided this to Joe, and he captured my enthusiasm to believe as only he can.

The next day was the one last ultrasound. I shouldn't have been surprised, I suppose, when the radiologist rubbed that gel on my belly and showed us that a cute little noggin was positioned where those ten little piggies had been waving just days before. I couldn't help tears of sweet relief. He had turned around. Upside down. Just like the song had said. Just as God had told me.

At first, the doctor was all for letting nature take its course from there and was a bit irked, I believe, that we wished to keep our scheduled appointment at the hospital. But as Joe had already arranged to be home from the road and was hoping he could go back to work, rushing his eighteen-wheeler from a state or two away in time for our little guy's impending arrival was just more stress than my fretful pregnant self could bear.

And so... mama was indulged, convenience was considered, and we merely switched gears from C-section to inducement, something I really never thought I'd be the sort to press for but was very grateful to have as a possibility in this crazy busy life we were living.

It was with that wild mix of anticipation and trepidation we set out that evening. I found myself duly gowned, stretched out with a warm cover to ward off that inevitable hospital chill, and hooked up to all those wires and monitors.

We sat for a timeless time just listening to the rapid whoosh of his tiny heartbeat, watching green lines etch themselves into a black screen. Up, down, up, down, up, down in a mostly monotonous pattern.

And then, I can remember a minor twinge or two. The green line shot up in a slight peak. The nurse uttered a slightly surprised *hmm* and turned to me to query, "Did you feel that?"

I sort of nodded, knowing there was no way it was a real contraction.

"Odd," she remarked.

It went on like that with only a very occasional pinch, much like what I had experienced heretofore, but not consistent. Not near enough to believe the little tyke might be helping the proceedings along.

And then they parked me in a room of my own, the room I was to give birth in, and discussed the need to soften my cervix. A bulb was to be placed inside me to facilitate this. A couple of interns and a nurse got me prepped and made the attempt, only to find it was already far too soft to even hold the bulb.

I was, in fact, still being administered the needed medicine to summon up labor, but as it so happened, David had somehow realized it was nearing his entrance time and had begun the exit process himself. Guided, naturally, by God's hand, the One who always had the timing on his eternal checklist written in stone.

So with very little coaxing, David John Ulrich wriggled out of the womb and into our hearts. Hungry, happy, and hearty. A little orange, and a little in need of Mr. Sun to flush the pumpkininess out, but otherwise in tip-top shape.

And he arrived at home like a little prince and swiftly found himself treated as such.

At almost ten and a half, just nine, and nearing eight, the older three were at terrific ages for appropriating the title of Mommy's Helpers. They fell right in with endearing attempts to entertain the baby, attacking their jobs of wipes hander and diaper fetcher with the utmost seriousness.

Don't want to sound like a Mary Sunshine, but I honestly can't recall an ounce of jealousy entering into the mix. Davey was much too much a novelty for any such struggle as that.

Proudly, they would parade through grocery stores and church, announcing for all to hear that tiny royalty was in the midst. And as he grew, so did their longing to teach him and equip him for kid life.

Not that there was never a tired nor a grouchy day. Certain tussles did continue. The Joe/Elijah battles over homework went on. The can't-do-its sometimes still cropped up in Sarah. The thunderous tears over mistakes found their way out of Timothy's sweet brown eyes at times. And me?

Well, I was tired, of course. Uncertain about embarking on this baby thing all over again and, at times, feeling a new chain in my one success at nursing.

And yet there was this blessed assurance that ran through the dinky halls of our little abode. There was a fondness in hearing childish voices voice the accents I once did in stories for them in stories they read for Davey. A smile and a glow and a wonder at getting to share these first giggles and roll-overs and scootings and a dozen other goings-on with a first-time dad. It made it new again for me, and I now had someone to call with the news of new teeth, new sounds, new delights when he was on the road and someone to sit close to on the couch and share news with when he got home.

And oh, the unadulterated joy that saturated me to know that Joe really, really wanted to be involved!

Holding Davey in church with a sweet daddy pride. Changing his diapers in spite of having to duck the spray. Coaxing him to try his sweet taters and green beans. It was so cool it was almost surreal to my do-it-myself personality. It'd really truly been that long since I'd experienced that side-by-side parenting as a unit thing. That lean in tight and help one another sense of family.

On one level, my parents, the older three, and I had certainly possessed a brand of it—a beautiful thing I will be forever grateful for. But there was something about this time of growing into parents and siblings and precious baby that was so special in its own right.

For a gurgly little piece of humanity was weaving an extra thread of togetherness in us all that served to unite us over hard times. Right there from his playpen. From the depths of his crib. The one that dominated our tiny bedroom floor space and caused dear Joe to have to climb over me to get out of bed. Unless I was dog-tired, I could count his every bathroom trip.

We looked around and could see the truth that wouldn't quit badgering us with every stuffed spot and stubbed toe. We had it all, but what we really needed was a bigger place for it all. But time and money and lack of credit as well as the ability to secure it seemed ever elusive.

And so here was yet another seemingly insurmountable obstacle at the outset that we found ourselves looking to the heavens to solve.

And the answer…well, it was just another case of all God…

Of course.

Chapter Eight
Where in the Heck is Pretty Prairie?

I was sitting on the couch, curled up in a throw as per usual on a cold January morn. Davey was practicing scooting around on his tummy time blanket, and the older three had been safely ushered to school.

It was a quiet time. A down time. In more ways than one.

We had recently been having discussions about Elijah, who was within months of wrapping up his elementary school years. He was grappling with more of that argumentative side than ever and starting to really feel that certain sting of identity search and a very real struggle with the work required.

Everyone involved with him at his current school was concerned, as we had been, with the question of where he'd be next year, how it'd work out, and whether he'd sink or swim.

For under that sometimes stridently oppositional side, we all knew an Elijah very dear to us, a sweet, well-meaning, and astonishingly smart and creative child we all feared might get lost in a large middle school atmosphere.

But stuck as we felt we were in our living situation, and as difficult as it already was to juggle transportation, I felt powerless to grasp a good possibility out of the confusing questions of what to do next.

It was in the midst of all this brooding that I picked up the local paper good ol' Mom graciously shared when she was done with her puzzles and picked through it.

Comics. Blah. Local and state. Further depression. Opinion page. Yeesh.

And then, just for laughs and daydreams, the classifieds.

Houses for sale. Gorgeous locales. Manicured lawns. Sturdy brick, best of schools, cream of the crop. Prices we could never aspire to reach unless Publisher's Clearinghouse came to our door with giant check and a fantastic flurry of balloons.

Big, heavy sigh from the depths of my pinned-down despair.

Davey gurgled nearby, contentedly chewing his rattle and nudging up new chompers, so young and with the good sense to be unaware there was more out there than this dinky apartment.

And here was I longing to nudge up new life when God had given so much already.

I shook my head in self-aggravated frustration and found my way back to reading. And it was then my eyes tripped down to it. Four or five-bedroom potential, two bath, owner carry, as is. Reasonable down payment and a monthly payment less than this sardine can we were currently squeezed into.

Wow. Now, that actually sounded like something. Lots of room. As is shouldn't be *too* big a deal with Joe's construction family upbringing, I think. Whoa, wait a minute…what's this?

In Pretty Prairie?

Pretty Prairie? Ummm…where is *that?*

I'd heard of a lot of the rinky-dink towns, fancy schmancy suburbs, and all things in between in Kansas by being both daughter and wife to truck drivers.

But never in my twenty-five years in the Sunflower state had I heard of Pretty Prairie.

I shrugged in defeat, figuring it had to be way out of the way and therefore not terribly reasonable in light of Joe's job, not to mention our families and church we weren't ready to pull up stakes from completely just yet.

The older three kids were still very much used to the frequent presence of grandparents in their lives. With them, routine had to be adjusted slowly.

Not to mention how welcome it was for us "trucker widows" to get together throughout the week. It would've proved much more lonesome some days otherwise.

But still, something in me *did* wonder. I had folded the paper over, but when I picked it back up, it fell right open to that ad again.

No. No. Stop dreaming.

Folded it over, laid it down again.

And yet…

Open to the ad once more.

I repeated this waffly little pattern twice before I just took a breath and decided to make the call.

To Joe. He was out in his truck. Surely, even if it had never come up in casual conversation before, he'd at least know where Pretty Prairie was.

Surprisingly, his recollection was only vague. Assisted by his trusty map, he finally let me know it was about forty minutes west of Wichita.

Not surprisingly, he sounded as intrigued as only a frustrated handyman disguised as a trucker could be. He requested the number and made the call.

And I researched my end: schools. Because we quickly reminded each other all of this would never even make it off the runway if the schools weren't right.

Amazingly, we both garnered positive responses fairly quickly. Both house and schools offered tours and seemed rather promising and accommodating.

And our parents all the way around sounded supportive. It was a bittersweet conversation to be sure, but they knew we needed to venture out and look for where life might be leading us, even if it wasn't just down the way from them.

And I began to see in my parents—particularly in Mom—the assurance that they thought the kids and I were indeed in capable hands. I felt I was growing into a more independent woman in my mom's eyes at long last.

We set out one morning when Joe had time away from the road—the school-agers at school, the little guy in his carrier, and the GPS firmly in place—and took a little road trip to see what we would see in this unknown blip on the map called Pretty Prairie.

We were both anxious and full of curious excitement as we neared the turn in the road that would bring us there.

Small could be cool. Small could be fun. Big house in a small town could be just what the doctor ordered.

We noted cute little places on the way in. Old and charming with porches that'd afford plenty of shade in summer. Vintage…just the way I liked it.

And then came the long dirt drive to the Main Street address from the ad.

And before us rose a really, really old home.

Large, gray, weathered. And I felt just a hint of trepidation steal into my excitement as we scooped up the carrier and opened the old white-painted door.

And stepped onto a wavy sea of puke green carpet that had caught and dried up from a whole lot of rain courtesy of the large and inconvenient hole in the roof, right smack over the middle of the living room.

Peely paint and plaster marred the walls everywhere. Two bedrooms and one bath were full of it.

The wave of carpeting continued into the dining room, and then there was the kitchen. Its one plus was its long stretch of cabinets, clear back to a little laundry alcove. *That* I could get with the program on.

However...

Inside, they were stinky and sticky and ringed with rusty spots where objects had once lived, and one or two were still stuffed with cans of cleansers—mostly unused—that were becoming permanent fixtures atop the dingy 1970-style shelf paper.

There was a stove somewhere under all the grease, I was sure, but whether it still worked was anyone's guess—there was no electricity or gas in this icebox to tell us.

Ah...call it vanity if you will, but for me, the house's major drawback of all drawbacks was the floor with a seven-layer cake of dirt and a yellowy frosting of age. It must've once been white. I was sure. But to bring it back to life?

I am no great housekeeper by any stretch—that's my mom, and I never reached for her heights—but I like for it to sort of look like I scrubbed the floor when I scrub the floor. And this was just to the point of impossible except by bulldozer.

We toured on to the basement. Oh, my! A dirty, freezing cold tomb. Large but largely unfinished. Peely wood paneling. Roots creeping out of the large closet in one room like a creature's claws groping for prey and boxes of abandoned stuff from times long past in another like some eerie museum display.

Looking around, that trepidation spreading like gangrene, I really felt myself shrink back and say inside, *No way is this our miracle.*

This was literally the house that time forgot.

And I glanced at my husband—ever the optimistic one when it came to such projects—and he was nodding his head, seemingly unperturbed by anything he was seeing, saying something along the lines of "We can do this."

I mumbled something doubtful as we disembarked from this Titanic of the Prairies and headed to check out the schools. There we were met with such sweetness, warmth, and promise, my heart felt a tug. They were small, homey, and quite likely beyond what I could hope for my dear young'ns.

We were graciously met by a very friendly secretary and the superintendent himself (doubling as grade school principal) who proved not too busy to take us around and reassure us of the good possibilities for *all* the kids—special needs and otherwise.

By the time the tour was done, my heart was being pulled all the more. Even the dismay of surveying the minuscule town itself with its lack of grocery, general store, or anything faintly resembling a McDonald's did nothing to diminish that sensation.

Made it maybe a little more troubled, but it was still there.

We climbed into the van and drove home a little less animatedly and a lot more thoughtful. Joe was no fool. He knew I was frightened, dismayed, and torn. He reiterated we could do it and described a bit of the how.

I nodded, taking it all in, but not completely. Honestly, my poor head was swirling madly as a host of things I did not fully understand about drywall and mudding and roof flashing and such came out of his mouth. Words I knew, but in a vocabulary I could really only guess the definitions of as one long stuck in the city, unused to anything but apartments, renting, and a dear dad who was a wonderful man but no handyman.

In the end, we agreed to pray about it, and pray I did—every spare moment I could find. It went something like this: *What do we doooo, Lord? What do we doooo? Want to help the kids, but is this spook house nightmare the way?* Nothing earthshattering, expansive, or full of faith-filled thee's and thou's. Actually, truth be known, it was rather whiny, weak, and whimpery.

But it got an answer.

Almost like a patient little nudge from Heaven.

Nothing ventured, nothing gained, I felt Him say.

I think I shocked Joe a bit when I said, "Let's do it," but he had already gathered long ago that if the kids could each have a room of their own and a decent school experience besides, those things would always outweigh any possible inconvenience.

So we took a deep breath, called the man, and put our hat in the ring along with two other interested parties.

And then we waited.

And waited.

And waited some more.

We'd been told the decision would be made in a couple of weeks, and we'd be informed either way. Two weeks had come and gone with nada. Part of me thought, *Well, there's the final answer. Just as well.* And yet...

I remember we were in the van, getting ready to unload all four kids and go do some grocery shopping, when something kept nagging at me. I mentioned the fact we hadn't heard anything and that maybe we should call so we'd know for sure if we should dismiss the whole idea and use our tax return money elsewhere.

Real positive stuff there.

Anyway...my nagging feeling passed on to Joe like a virus, and he picked up his cell with a bit of irritation and dialed the guy's number.

I can still remember the excitement flooding from the tiny speaker up to Joe's ear and clear over to mine. I couldn't make out all the words, but from what I *could* get, this man was absolutely thrilled we'd called. A believer himself, he'd prayed hard about what he ought to do. God had told him to give the property to us and to knock off a thousand from the down payment besides.

But the kicker was this—he'd lost our number! He had been praying about how to get back in touch with us when Joe called.

Okay, God, I thought. *I can't walk away from this one.* Another case of orchestration from the greatest of conductors.

I guessed it was time to figure out how to use a hammer and live in the sticks…all at the same time.

Chapter Nine
Greeeeen Acres Is...the Place To...Be?

And so work began in that frosty February.

Work in unheated, unwatered, unbelievably filthy quarters.

Every day Joe could get home from the road, we were there. Managing busted old water lines, fighting messed-up old gas lines, sifting through trash of yesteryear and probably that of a few party animals past.

Judging, examining, purchasing.

Tarring and decking and roofing.

Well, beyond the cleaning, it was just about all Joe. My not-afraid-to-get-his-hands-knuckle-deep-in-dirt hero.

My job most days went like this: Praying and crying and jiggling Davey and figuring out what I could clean till the water could get turned on (not much).

And then, there was worry on my shoulder as Joe tied on a safety rope and climbed up on the roof all by his—don't get me wrong—*very* capable but somehow so vulnerable self to tear off and reshingle this sad, tired Green Acres clone.

So I prayed some more. Found us dismayed by snow. By cantankerous delays in gas lines, water lines, and so on, and so on. And then I sat down and felt infinitely alone in this struggle, though I knew deep down it wasn't so.

Mom and Dad came out some, too, pitching in where they could, trying and failing and trying some more to be encouraging, laying a hand to things they had never done, fetching supplies they were highly unused to purchasing when we were in our rental home and apartment, living a nonhandy existence.

PaPa Orbie—he fixed things. Well, jerry-rigged sometimes, but he knew the ins and outs of a hardware store. But *my* folks? Well, it wasn't a concern in our world most days. So...there was a lot of "Huh?" and "What?" and "How do I find/do that?" to much of the stuff Joe rattled off in his expertise.

And it seemed like every day there was something more to buy, eating up the tax return money at an alarmingly rapid pace for penny pincher me.

I tried not to fret, tried to give it all to God like I knew I should. I listened to our portable CD player sing out songs of praise while I sat in that cold tomb, but looking around—while I knew there was internal progress as well as amazing strides being made on the roof between latent spring snows—it was still so ugly inside to me.

Barren. Warpy carpeted. Stained. Moldy (went through gallons of bleach fending off that one).

I felt lazy, incompetent even. Taking an eyesore and making it a home just wasn't in me, I feared. It wasn't that I expected a finished product handed to me on a silver platter—my life had taught me way too much to buy into that lie. No, it was almost as though that reserve of strength that'd carried me so far for so long had all but dried up. Every day we trekked from our cozy little Wichita abode to this house that time forgot, I grew crankier and more resentful. Almost hopeless.

Joe, for his part, kept on. I could see the stress weighing on his shoulders, edging into his voice as we discussed our various hurdles on any given day as well as the fact that extra hands to help seemed sparse most weeks, despite repeated pleas to our church family. We tried not to let it get us too down, though a shadow began to fall over some relationships there. A shadow I wasn't ready to examine too closely.

And then, of course, work was tugging hard at him as well, expecting more and further runs despite his adamant wishes to be at home more. My grumpies and his worries fed off each other, and it wasn't a pretty sight.

One day, tinkering away at this really old house, Joe's curiosity got up. He'd been working on something on the lower level—I forget what as there were so many tasks that they all tangled in my mind like so many knots—when he noted something above that seemed like wood that just might be the floors above.

Quick as a wink, he was charging up the icky old basement stairs, peeling back the nasty green vomit carpet for a peek, motioning me over with an explanation to have a look with him.

First, we spied subfloor, but then, after his pry bar broke some of that loose, nothing but black.

Oh. My heart dropped in disappointment. I hadn't even realized it'd lifted at the idea of hardwood floors, but it had.

And then, he began to peel the black, too.

Much to my surprise, there was a fairly gleaming bit of oak winking up at me!

"It's probably all over the house," Joe remarked. "Protected by tar paper for who knows how many years."

And my abandoned hope found flight once more.

Over our next few project days, I dug in harder than I ever had, my vigor renewed by this new task of ripping up yucky carpet, loosening subfloor, and tearing up tar paper to find my shiny wooden prize beneath.

I'd always dreamt of hardwood floors, you see, through all the years of the crunchy, hopeless beige carpets of my first marriage and my single mom years.

The ones that were swiftly stained despite my best efforts. The ones that screamed failure up at me and chided me for how I'd mismanaged Elijah and the Kool-Aid over here and allowed a potty-training incident to occur over there.

And those things always happened when I was stuck home and tapped out on carpet cleaner—when I could afford it at all, that is.

This possibility of something I'd longed for so much and for so long was like a nudge from above, a reminder He was in this whole thing yet.

Chagrined at small faith, I whispered my heartfelt thanks, cranked up the praise music, and sang louder than I'd dared in so long.

This was going to be a good place, I decided. A life-changing place. A place where sweat and perseverance would bring out beautiful results.

The results of yet more hopes and dreams long deferred coming to pass.

God even showed me clearly in this time that one day, there would be ministry flowing out of this property, as well as in the two old airplane hangars behind us. Youth would be pulled from the bored and restless streets to our door to learn something valuable—both in electrical trade and in a redeemed life in Christ.

Joe would teach, I would feed, and this house would be a hub for change.

It was a lofty dream, one neither of us could fully comprehend in the here and now nor put away. So, like Mary, I had yet more to treasure in my heart as we moved ahead with plans.

We tackled a good many necessary projects in those coming weeks. Floors, roof, walls began to come under relative control.

We were shooting for a move in late May—the end of the school year, the end of our beginnings in Wichita. All was feeling bittersweet and nostalgic and possible.

The kids were adjusting to the move as well, the more we talked about it. There was the understandable, undeniable sorrow of leaving familiar places and people behind, but excitement at the adventure and the elbow room to come.

It was still backbreaking work, to be sure. But there was such a sense of destiny to it all, and we were all beginning to get caught up in the enthusiasm despite the heartaches.

And then, that April day came when Joe trudged home from a long. tough run.

With every bit of what he normally kept in his truck.

He'd been let go, along with fifteen other drivers that preferred regional runs that got them home at least once a week.

And it felt as though the bottom had dropped out one more time.

Chapter Ten
Electrical Dreams,
Unemployment Realties,
and Reasons for Faith

Our first fears were, of course, how we would make it. Take care of the kids. The bills. The house. How would we sustain this move, *could* we sustain this move, would we lose everything we'd been working so incredibly hard for?

We'd already turned in our thirty-day notice to our landlord. They were already actively seeking new renters. Turning back didn't seem like a feasible or desirable option.

Or faith-filled.

And so, as a family, we swiftly made the decision to trust that the God who landed this house for us would bring about the right work at the right time.

In the meantime, there was still a bit of that tax return left to hold us over while Joe looked for work.

We were quickly reminded of two things in his search: there are few trucking companies that want their employees putting family as a top priority and even fewer places that don't frown on a history that includes nine years in Lansing, albeit youthful years long past and covered under the impeccable blood of Jesus.

It was soon a discouraging venture, this job search, but one we felt was meant to launch Joe in an area removed from trucking and more suited to his new family, his natural skills, and his desires.

When nothing was panning out, he began to look into his long-ago dreams of electrical work. He'd nearly completed school for this years ago, hindered only at the last by a stolen truck and no offers for transportation to class.

The union looked promising, and apprenticeship was an actual possibility pending approval and passing of tests. Money would be great from the looks of the brochures. Maybe, maybe this was the answer all along!

So we charged ahead with the move.

Facing further disappointment with returning mold, we found ourselves tearing down panels just recently put up to finish the kids' walls in the basement.

I admit there were tears at that for me, but we surged forward with the bright hope that one day, Joe would be an official electrician, and all our plans for beautifying this place could become reality.

So things got boxed and transported, and when we ran out of boxes, things got tossed in backseats and bags and baskets. A few faithful church friends came and whipped some things into shape for us.

And then, they just about unraveled us with an impromptu scolding about Joe's smoking. Tempers flared. I played chicken to their pressure and didn't defend him. I will never forget that sad feeling of surrendering to someone else's harsh judgment yet again, nor the sharp dagger of division it slices through a husband and wife.

Not a proud moment in this whole getting-together-as-a-family adventure. It was as if the devil was trying one last, nasty swipe to bring us down before this very purposeful move, and the ones who had meant well with their assistance had only caused that shadow I was feeling about our church to grow darker.

The results of my not standing by him were swift. There was injurious betrayal in his eyes, anger rising up at being, for all intents and purposes, under attack for something he had yet to be able to conquer in a long list of things he'd conquered in life. And I felt that old fear that someone would leave me rise up inside.

Before he was set to drive off in the moving truck with me to follow behind in my mom's car, I ran to him. Bawling and unashamed in front of friends and family, I ran.

And felt silly...but still spilled out my profuse apologies, relieved to receive his forgiveness. It was a moment that could've served to tear us apart but wound up being a chance to mend.

That vitally important piece secured once more, we were on our way.

Out of Wichita. Out of the old lives. Into the new and the unknown. And hopeful that despite all bumps, this new would promise to be better than anything we'd ever known.

* * *

Settling in took, obviously, a fair amount of time for this family of six plus one furry baby. The realization swiftly sunk in that we, forced by finances and time shortage, were indeed moving the three older kids into a basement with eerily cavelike features, including mostly bare walls in need of drywall, paint, and cheeriness and cold cement floors.

About the time we started unloading and arranging, *I* started unloading apologies to them for the unfinished state of being, followed by desperate avowals this was all temporary, that one day, Daddy would be a well-off electrician, and we'd have funds enough to make their rooms whatever they could dream up.

It was funny, though, how little they complained. In fact, despite my and my mother's oh-my-goodness-three of-our-babies-are-sleeping-down-*there* mentality, the kids were just eager to spread out and start having fun in their new, much-expanded digs. I have always said give them a plain box and their imagination, and they'll come up with a thousand games.

I just never pictured that plain box would be three terribly plain rooms.

Or that I'd once again find myself humbled from my depressed, grouchy state by my own children.

Soon we found ourselves getting into a certain groove, tackling more projects as we could, exploring the new delights of summer in a country town, frequenting low-cost amusements like strolls to the library, running in the humongous yard, attending the wonderful free movies shown every week at the cool old-fashioned theater.

If the kids were bored, they rarely let on. If they were fretful Dad was home so much of the time—other than a few weeks when, thankfully, he had an opportunity to participate in a harvest and bring home that wondrous thing called money—they never said. In fact, they just enjoyed.

For promise of a new future was coming. We just had to keep stepping forth. All would be well in time, we assured ourselves.

Joe still checked into every possibility he thought might propel him forward in this dream of being an electrician, but really, I think we all pressed a lot of weight on that hopefully impending apprenticeship.

And then, Joe's final exam came and went with that continued confidence. Everyone involved seemed impressed with his natural knowledge and passion. We were sure a resounding yes was on its way from Wichita to Pretty Prairie, straight to our orange-red-blue (painted based purely on the older kids' favorite colors) mailbox.

We continued traveling weekly to our church there in Wichita, and they helped pour the enthusiasm and prayer on even more.

Destiny was the catch phrase, and caught it we did.

So when the letter came, dear Joe opened it with eager, shaky hands. Here was destiny…but what we read threw us for quite a loop.

He had passed the exam quite well, but an apprenticeship could not be offered. He lacked the 450 hours of job experience required, but this fact had never been disclosed to him till that point.

Many surprised and borderline frantic calls were made in those days, attempts made to find out why this information was not handed out from the get-go, what his recourses were, where he might obtain this experience, and so on.

There were few answers to satisfy. No companies in the area were willing to hire outside the union. There was no one to give him this coveted, needed start. No way to get a foot in the door to what we all assumed *was* the foot in the door. A real catch-22 if ever there was one.

And later, by others in the know, it was intimated that it's really about having a good sponsor on the inside of the union. Sadly, another case of *who* you know and not necessarily always *what* you know.

So...it was back to a case of what now? How would the future look? How would we feed, clothe, and keep a roof over the kids' heads, much less give the rest of this half-finished house shape?

I pondered my own possibilities in this time, but frankly, in this town of one gas station, zero stores, and families that mostly took care of their own kiddos and grandkiddos, no viable opportunities arose. Add to that issues of increased joint pain, transportation concerns, making enough to do more than feed the babysitter, as well as just that natural pull to be home, keep nursing Davey, and be present for the older kids left it rather unfeasible.

We had unemployment, but it wasn't much considering the six people it was supposed to sustain. Yet, in gratitude, we stretched it as far as possible for quite a time.

One summer twilight, we met a couple while taking a stroll and started chatting. Before long, they took it upon themselves to become substitute mother and father where ours could not be physically at that present time.

Word spread, food poured in, clothing rained down, and providence started to peek through in most unexpected ways.

The unpayable somehow got paid. The impossible somehow got toppled. We even once received one of those fabled mailbox miracles—addressed to us from us—containing two hundred dollars. (Just after I'd jokingly said it'd be nice to get one before Joe went to check the mail, I might add. God just loves a sense of humor!) And we began to see, through it all, that this Pretty Prairie was more than just a pretty prairie. There were actual real, kind, loving, generous neighbors. Christians who believed in swift, kindly action more than half-hearted prayers.

It was another case of humbling circumstance for me, shy and reluctant as I was, that others who barely knew us yet were so willing to see to our need.

It was quite the challenge to let go and simply allow God to use them as vessels for such. Yet in the midst of this often shaky period, my heart could not help but soar at such happenings as well as at the providence and protection we kept running into right and left.

I still remember the first big hailstorm that summer. It rushed through our little town like a speeding freight train, pelting windows and roofs and vehicles unmercifully, its fierce gales taking out a great deal of the interiors of the few buildings on our main street, including the beloved theater we'd been enjoying in those early months of exploration.

Naturally, the kids and I had scooted down to the basement fairly quickly. Joe had that family protector's instinct to remain upstairs to watch the proceedings for a bit. I didn't exactly like it, but if I'd learned one thing about my husband, it was to leave aside argument when he is determined.

So...I huddled up with my precious babes there on the bathroom tile, Davey nestled in my lap, and prayed. We had been in the house maybe two months. I can admit to a pretty sizable chunk of fear that all might be lost as the wind whipped like a madman around us. More than that, of course, I feared for Joe's safety.

It was not one of those profound, faith-filled prayers, but you have probably gathered by now that those are few and far between with me. It was more like a stomach-churning cry: "Please, God, please, I'm so scared! Please keep us safe! Protect my husband! Protect this house! We just got it! Don't let us lose it!"

The wildness of it all didn't last long, though. Soon enough, I could hear no more from beyond the basement windows. As Joe's steps sounded on the stairs, I let out the breath I never realized I was holding. I couldn't help reaching out to cling to his sleeve in relief.

As I tugged at him, he crouched beside us with wide eyes, and I could see something had him stirred. He was rarely like this.

In breathless tones, he began to describe something that astounds me yet. He'd been standing there, looking through the front door at the chaos, praying as I'd been praying for the protection of the house and his family.

All of a sudden, the solid mass of rain and hail driving down from every direction parted! He could glance to the right and still see one sheet, to the left and see another. But our property? Well, the hail was hurling *away* from it rather than toward as it'd just been a moment before!

All told, though, sadly, other homes and buildings saw more extensive damage. When we surveyed the house after, only three storm windows had suffered some cracks, and the garage roof Joe was set to have to tear off and redo anyway had been swept clean for him. But not a shingle from the new house roof he'd labored over those many months had so much as stirred.

Neighbors all over were agog as we all pitched in to pick up limbs the next few days. All we could really say was, "That's God."

Yet more staggering proof that He fully intended us to be here. And it was amazing how many folks came out of the woodwork to warmly agree. Joe, in particular, was allowed to demonstrate his best helper mode here, and we began to find a delightful give and take too few communities have these days.

We felt as though we had certainly found one of the few God-fearing places left in the country. Oh, sure, Pretty Prairie had—and has—its share of party people, and a few who are reluctant about Jesus, but there was and is such an openness about genuine faith that shines through in a very refreshing way.

We had seen it before the storm, of course, and it was even present at our first ever rodeo which fell just right for Timbo's ninth birthday and provided the beginnings of a grand tradition. It was filled with more than just cowboy hats, mechanical bulls, and excitement. It began with heartfelt prayer. But somehow, after the storm, with all the damage assessed, we felt a tighter kinship. We were fellow survivors. In this together.

And, dare I say, in the humblest way, we were providing testimony to His goodness. The bare beginnings of a lighthouse to this small, struggling place?

Certainly, all this gave us courage as we pressed on to grapple with the never-ending task of caring for our family.

One church, in particular, began to shine brightly in that time, for they seemed determined to extend more than just a hand and opened the doors for the older three kids' first VBS (Davey was young yet for it all, not even quite a year, but already so watchful of everything the big kids did, I knew he'd one day be enthused for such).

I was excited for this opportunity for the kids to hopefully meet future classmates, but naturally, mixed in there was a nervous nelly of a special needs mom, protective and worried about how well this would go over.

Would they do or say something incomprehensible?

Would they cry?

Be stand-offish?

Unable to master the games?

Tongue-tied about bathroom communication?

So much any mom thinks about, I know, but my tape played in blaring stereo.

To my complete surprise, with a little information on their sides about my precious babes, the teachers couldn't say enough about how terrific the kids did, how delightful they were.

Elijah was deemed quiet but studious and creative. Timothy, sweet, smart, and enthusiastic. Sarah, joyful, friendly, and light-hearted.

All those things we as parents knew day by day and only hoped others would or could see.

* * *

And then, all at once, time rushed forward as it does, and the first school year arrived, and somehow the kids had clothes, supplies, and a ready spirit for it all. Teachers and paras and therapists were at the ready as well. Each one swift on the uptake, prepared and communicative for the most part. Just the way I liked and needed it.

All the while, adoption of the older three by Joe had been in the works as well. We rejoiced that my ex-husband made the sacrifice to sign over parental rights, stipulating only that he might continue to visit with the three when convenient.

Blessedly, it had been paid for in a time when money was present. God again seeing to the need.

It was such a sweet victory to see the final papers after all those months of wrangling, the birth certificates, all of it in print with the name Ulrich on it, the father Joseph. At last, we were all officially under one umbrella.

The kids, my in-laws, Joe, and I celebrated with dinner and certificates, courtesy of my ever-talented and lovely mother-in-law, and with lots of pictures showcasing wide grins.

The kiddos had never really expressed anything but fondness for their biological dad. Maybe some deep down hints of wistfulness at wanting things to be different, wanting him to want them more, wanting to see him and their half-siblings more, and, compassionate kids that they are, wishing for me to not have had my years of sadness. But as to anger, it just didn't seem to bubble up in any sort of verbal display.

Yet that day, just as our wedding day, was such a heart-soaring, being chosen kind of feeling. Someone wanted us. *All* of us. Someone went through quite a lot of money, time, and effort to ensure this kind of forever. There was no doubt about the joy in that moment for everyone.

So yes, we were well underway in many, many things...yet still scrambling in others. Joe had at last secured a job that fall, only to have it unfairly snatched away two months after.

Now, I honestly hadn't been in love with this opportunity due to the grueling schedule, but we figured beggars couldn't be choosers, and steady income after a long, desert-dry period was welcome relief, so this sudden, extremely cruel turn of events was, frankly, rather mixed for me, though the anger at encountering yet another catch-22 situation, not to mention seeing my beloved rather violently blackballed just because he outperformed his superiors, won out for a time over any relief I might've had.

We had unwittingly discovered an ominous side to this area where towns are small, the pool of work possibilities smaller, and justice sometimes takes a backseat to lifelong drinking buddies.

For a time, I was in full-on crusade mode, writing letters and sharing the story so others might get stirred as well. Upon discovering Kansas is a right-to-work state, meaning it is completely at the employer's discretion to let an employee go for any whim, and learning our only other recourse was a long, potentially expensive lawsuit, we bowed out and tried hard to find God's grace in it all.

The third shift hours and every other Sunday *had* been miserable in short order. The sense of family was slipping through our fingers, church in Wichita was relegated to every other week, and those things which we had fought to start smoothing out between us, between Joe and the kids, were getting rumpled again as time and tired crankiness had taken over.

I honestly can look back now and see it was a case of God working it all together for good. Reminding us we must set our eyes on Him and Him alone.

For everything.

There was a little unemployment yet in reserve and the very occasional back child support Billy owed yet. My folks were in the middle of upheaval in their own right, moving to my grandparents' long empty home in Oklahoma after much persuading by my dear uncle who had been caring for my mentally ill aunt on his own ever since Granny and PaPa had passed.

He needed respite, and they needed a change.

In this series of transitions, this was a really, really hard one. It'd been hard enough to be in a different city. An era was officially ending where Mom and Dad were always just a small drive away, next to us on Sunday mornings, present for hugs and visits, and available for advice and giggles on McDonald's afternoons.

But even in the midst of our chaos, it was time. They exhibited the trust the Lord and my Joe had rightfully earned, signaled they knew, in spite of it all, we'd be all right, and went to be where life could be rent-free, legacies could live on, and a tired man could get two extra pairs of shoulders to carry some of the burden.

It was all so bittersweet, indeed.

Before long, Thanksgiving and Christmas loomed large, and with them, obviously, the where, the when, the how would it all come together with the tiny pittance the state offered, few prospects of work in sight, and hope stretching sorrowfully threadbare despite all efforts to hold fast to God.

For Thanksgiving, we wound up scraping together gas enough to travel to Oklahoma to help christen the old house anew with my folks. There was comfort in those old walls, relief at seeing the house in a more righted state than when I'd last visited my grief-stricken, fragile-as-a-bird PaPa, and an odd sort of different sameness at being there.

It was almost as if I could hear Granny's old hymns pouring out in the hum of the place, girding us and guiding us ever to the old rugged cross for another helping of amazing grace, blessed assurance alongside it.

There was joy mingled with the grief, a joy that comes only in knowing salvation is ever present, providence's promise is ever on its way, and the spirits of those gone on before us continue to rest within us, participating with us and cheering us on as a piece of that cloud of witnesses that just *knows* that with God, all things are possible.

We left with many tender prayers, hugs, wishes, and food boxed up with love, leaving our folks with at least the comfort that, thus far, we were sustained. Thus far, the schools were awesome. Thus far, the community was welcoming.

And then, we came home. To a Christmas we still knew not how to prepare for. We'd received so much from our folks without being able to give much in return. We knew, of course, there was no stopping a grandparent from giving, but we were determined to not drain them dry.

With equal parts surrender and dismay, we set out to keep it all very simple and homemade yet loving and caring. I would try my hand—and try not to stab it—at sewing dolls though I was by no means a seamstress. We would compile CDs of wonderful Christian music for our music lovers. Joe would build a big red box to hold all Elijah's precious origami, comics, and the like.

We would not worry about ourselves because sometimes parents just have to do that. And it was okay. We loved one another, and we knew it, and God loved us, and we knew that, too. It would be enough. Oh, how we prayed it'd be enough.

I don't know if it was just that the decision we'd reconciled ourselves to make pleased God's heart or if we'd just forgotten He might have different plans. Whatever it was, something came along to bowl us over and cement the realization that the eyes of the Lord and the eyes of this community were ever upon us—to love us and to bestow a bounty upon us. A Christmas spirit that overshadows all, courtesy of that humble babe in the manger we sing all the songs about and too often forget to attribute miraculous happenings to.

Chapter Eleven
Belief Rebuilt, and Basement to Come

I will never forget that first phone call. Someone I'd yet to meet had somehow secured our names and wanted to know all the basics about our kiddos—ages, sizes, fondest pursuits, and Christmas dreams. They wanted to put them on a community angel tree. Another instance of finding out that this really, really is how this little town rolls.

We'd had a taste, of course, but I don't know if we promptly forgot or perhaps, more likely, we hadn't wanted to lean this much upon relative strangers in this our first Christmas season in the new home.

Charity is a wondrous thing, but it's hard to keep asking for it and equally hard to take. Especially for us do-it-yourself types. Joe had been able to pitch in a bit after the storm, but we were heavy yet with the burden of obligation to repay what had already been poured out to us.

She'd called Joe first, but he'd wisely directed her to me, resident keeper of all such information.

So it was with a startled and uncertain heart that I began to list for her all I could in matters of sizes and needs. And then we got to those wondrous things that make the kids who they are— Timothy's voracious reading appetite, Elijah's building prowess, Sarah's sparkly princess personality, David's sturdy growth and penchant for all things with wheels.

And something joyous clicked in me. Gratitude. And I thanked her profusely and hung up the phone and discussed it all with Joe with grins and childlike enthusiasm and praise to a God always looking out for us.

Almost like I was six again and skipping along in the midst of Christmas cheer.

But we found it wasn't over yet. Soon we were fielding several more calls. Someone wanted to give us a deep freeze. Another dear lady who had lost her grown son years before and had no grandchildren to spoil was looking to spoil ours. And the food— oh, the food! Our big long line of kitchen cabinets could scarcely contain it all.

And then came the cream of the crop. A sweet couple from the church the kids attended VBS at wanted to come by with gifts one evening. They presented to us a basket overflowing with bounty. Conversation was lovely, effusive, and so full of God I could feel His presence weighty in the room. Sometimes there are just those connections with other Christians that are so immediate it blows you away. That was how it felt that night. And then came a card.

The card. The gentleman had passed it to Joe as head of the family and instructed him to open it. The front was a warm, lovely mix of red and gold with kind Christmas wishes inscribed that Joe read aloud in his broad, deep tones. Inside…

Well, inside was a personal note that Joe only got midway through reading before choking up and passing it to me, unable to finish. It wasn't often I'd had the privilege of seeing such. But seeing what was written there, I quickly surmised why, as my own voice filled with tears, and I stumbled through the words: a $2600 collection had been taken and volunteers gathered to help finish the kids' rooms.

I still well up today in memory as I write this.

How? we marveled. *How could this be?* Nobody knew. Nobody had inquired. We sure hadn't advertised the fact the basement was a dreary, nasty tomb and that it would have to remain that way until we could afford all it would need to be transformed, or just how much it saddened our hearts to realize that.

And then we recalled while we were in Enid visiting at Thanksgiving, the first dear couple we'd met in town had offered to keep a key to our place for emergency's sake. They had called one day while we were gone to report a light on in the basement and asked if we wanted them to go turn it off.

Of course was what we'd said at the time. Not really remembering leaving it on, but not really puzzling too hard on it all the same.

On this December evening, it came into focus. There were fantastic, lovely, sneaky little elves roaming our basement while we ate leftover turkey and reminisced with my mom and dad. Measurements were taken, assessments were made, estimates were duly noted and generously supplied for.

All because we had taken a moment one of those early summer nights to speak to someone new.

You just really, really never know how one small event piles upon another and leads to those desires of your heart finding sweet fulfillment.

We ended that night with such humble thankfulness and blessed prayer. Plans to tinker away at these brand new rooms were set for January. We went to bed that night in such awe of His goodness. How could we ever doubt?

* * *

A few days before Christmas saw a fresh flood of giving as the gifts purchased for the kids poured in. So many glossy packages and twinkly bags we hardly knew where to stow them at first. Until we recalled the big box Joe had crafted for Elijah. We hauled it into our bedroom, filled it up to the brim, and threw some blankets over top to lessen suspicions and curiosity.

When we sent the kids to bed Christmas Eve, what fun it was to pull it all out and spread it about under the tree. It was definitely a case of cups and trees running over. Joe decided to put the tree on top of the box and use it to pile some of this incredible bounty on.

That morning, the wonder in their eyes was gift enough for me. To watch them—gratefully rather than greedily—tear into package after package was just beautiful. There were even a couple for me and Joe, but it was just sprinkles on the icing of this delightful cake. The real joy was in seeing our kids—who mostly knew Santa was just an endearing myth—see providence at work. And real-life Christians living out life the way Jesus said to. Fine, worthy lessons I so longed to teach them and never expected them to learn in this humbling, miraculous way.

The close of that year made so much more seem possible.

And then, that January, we saw that so much more both come to be and seem to elude all over again.

Chapter Twelve
Help! Is There a Heavenly Handyman in the House?

January saw a busy flurry of things. Groups of men from the Mennonite church who'd extended the amazingly generous offer assembled to begin the work on the basement with ladies right behind to provide the food to feed the hearty crew.

It was all wondrous and overwhelming—shifting things out of the kids' rooms and opening my highly imperfect home to (don't get me wrong) very, very kind people but people I still only knew vaguely at best. It was hard for the likes of shy, retiring me.

Part of the issue was that in my experience, people were nice till they weren't nice anymore, and some of them, sadly, had been church people. While I could celebrate this present kindness with utter gratitude, under there was such self-consciousness, a reluctance to fully open myself, and an undeniable desire to run and hide from all things social for fear of the looming judgment.

I felt rather guilty to have such thoughts when God had been so good, but there they were.

After all these years and all the healing that'd taken place in my heart and in my life, I felt myself shrinking back into those age-old struggles. I was chagrined to see I really could only do small surface things like a hello in passing, a hint of conversation on the street, a thank you for the beautiful blessings. That I could only believe the best of them on a limited basis.

Only so long as my real self with holes enough to rival Swiss cheese didn't get found out.

So...the low-esteem me was honestly in paradox to the one so grateful for all that was going on in our midst. I silently counted the hours till the work days were over and thanked the Lord not just for the progress, but also for the peaceful quiet that reigned after.

And yet, here and there, there were those opportunities sprinkled in, meant to stretch me, and as I related our lives and times to the women who took turns providing delicious dinners, I slowly learned that our story really did bless others. The fact that somebody might be genuinely interested kind of blew me away. Not for gossip or untold condescending thoughts, I marveled. But…for love of God and fellow man.

It wasn't like it was the first time anyone had been good to me. There was, after all, our Wichita church. While that little shadow of concern about our longtime place of worship sometimes still peeked through from time to time, I loved the people of the church dearly and was not quite ready to let go. True, there was a certain amount of strain now that we were not conveniently close, and hands there didn't often extend in this practical way we were seeing in Pretty Prairie, but they were family. And we were *told* the spirit of God was moving there. Sometimes I even felt it yet.

I found myself treasuring it all in my heart in a deeper way than I ever had before. Despite my usual, distrustful tendencies, it was such a joy to watch our lives unfold in this new way. It was almost funny to say I longed for more of the camaraderie this church seemed to possess to feel further from our own.

However, there was no time to analyze much in the realm of receiving because, in addition to all being rebuilt in our home, something else began to build up around this time, something that would drastically change our family's direction and expand our vision that much further.

* * *

A well-dressed gentleman approached the house one day that winter, I recall. Unemployment was tapped out, jobs were meager, and hope was becoming just as thin as a weak broth, and, at times, just as nourishing. Where we saw so much cheer beginning in the basement, this area of our lives was still rather downcast.

Answering the queries about work week after week with, "No, not yet" was wearing on us all. Looking into the increasingly wondering eyes of our children was sinking my heart. My "not today" reply to the simple things they wanted at times had become more than I could bear.

So when this well-to-do man, introducing himself as a brother-in-law to the dear gentleman we were purchasing the house from, stepped up onto our dusty old porch and asked to speak with Joe about work, we were definitely more than just intrigued.

Word had gotten round to him that Joe was a handyman of sorts and that pounding the pavements had brought little but worn feet and holey shoes. He proposed hiring him out at a fair hourly wage to remodel two properties he'd recently purchased. We were instantly encouraged that this could keep him busy a while and, perhaps, launch something lasting.

Now, he couldn't have known this had long been Joe's dream—to run his own remodel and repair business. I hadn't even fully known. Oh sure, he'd batted it around with me a time or two, but honestly, I hadn't known just how deep it ran till that day.

We all, of course, found great relief at the thought of steady money, but there was, beyond that, a boyish glow dancing in Joe's eyes that spoke volumes. Something he loved to do, and the offer to be paid to do it? Be still his construction-working heart. Be still my wifely pride.

And thus, Heavenly Handyman was born out of equal parts long-held desire and desperate need.

Of course, it wasn't an official moniker in those days. It remained more a thought than anything then. For, of course, one job did not a business make. But oh, it was a job! At long last!

So Joe plunged in with both feet, shrewdly assessing needs, examining materials and advising purchases, outlining what would need to be done to bring these properties into rental-worthy shape.

His upbringing in all things building really shone, and overall, this, his first client, really seemed to radiate enthusiasm in the beginning months. Trust was fairly readily given as this man had a home in North Carolina and an extensive travel schedule to keep. He kept tabs via phone calls, but for the most part, Joe was free to do the work on a fairly flexible if steady basis. What a wonderful setup for a do-it-himselfer and dad of four often needed at home at odd times for an appointment here or an IEP there!

I can admit that aspect of it was pure bliss. No more fretting for this vehicularly challenged lady, nor for the mama who sometimes just really, really wanted that involved sort of daddy for her very own.

All began to move along a little less bumpily for a time. There was a concern or two arising about Elijah and the daunting tasks of middle school, but nothing I felt a little more communication and understanding wouldn't solve. He had a teacher who was always looking for ways to do that—from assignments of origami and comics for the class paper to opportunities rich with do-overs. So I worried, but I didn't. At least, not any more than usual.

Overall, these were busy days but peaceful days. A sense of accomplishment at long last days. A sense of having enough to tend to our needs days.

But as the first of the two houses began to wrap up that spring, there was a growing unrest. Less agreeableness spewed forth in those phone calls from North Carolina to Kansas. Hints of tightfistedness and unwillingness to do right by the properties and future renters rose up to taint the atmosphere with worry and frustration. Many an evening, Joe came home with a lot less tired satisfaction and a lot more just plain tiredness. He was tired of phone-wrangling, being second-guessed, and being put-off. Tired of a man who couldn't seem to trust him as he'd done in the beginning, a man who changed his mind more often than the designer clothing he always wore.

I sat by and tried to listen without my typical fretfulness creeping in. I tried to pray for his patience and for a return to those all-too-brief days of surety we'd enjoyed. It was clear the work Joe wanted to do to right this second house and the work the man was willing to fund were two different things. And where the first house had needed mostly touchups (except for some attention it ought to have received in Joe's eyes and did not till long after the renter had suffered multiple floodings), this second house was on par with our *Green Acres* nightmare. Only a total gutting would bring it to rights, and it wasn't something Joe would or could do in a slapdash fashion. His integrity wouldn't allow him.

I admit I had enormous pride in that, mixed with the worry of losing the first real income we'd had in so long. Where a teensy piece of me asked, "Couldn't you just ride it out?" a bigger part of me knew that was the question that would really make or break him.

As husband, as dad, as business owner.

As a man of God.

So when my husband came home with the news his client no longer had funds to pay for the venture and had attempted to attack his work ethic, all the while maintaining no true concept of ever having him do it correctly, I knew this particular job was done.

Again? My heart sighed a bit. And yet...we had business cards now. And word of mouth to carry us. That fierce tigress of anger snarled a bit at yet another person doing my beloved husband wrong, but God calmed it swiftly with reminders to hold onto the gratitude for the chance this man had given to launch Joe's dreams.

For this was still only the beginning. The town believed in him, supported his integrity and sense, and was beginning to see the quality of his work was every bit as high as promised.

Our Wichita church prayed with us even though we feared they were fatigued by our requests.

Mom and Dad made the trek up from Oklahoma to watch over the kids to give us a brief but needed respite. Stress was wearing us down more than either of us wanted to admit in those days, fraying our nerves and weighing on our patience with one another.

It's hard to realize that even among we who so fiercely fight to defend the God-given, miracle-cultivated ground so precious to us, time and trying circumstances can darn near defeat you. So when financial breakthrough appeared, and we had the opportunity to attend a Marriage Encounter weekend, we leaped on it. I was thrilled by the fact I didn't have to beg Joe to go. He was as sensitive to the Spirit as a wife could hope for, recognizing as well as I that we were sorely in need. It was a tentative start with so much writing and sharing involved I feared Joe might shut down or bolt from being so out of his element, but the more we pressed forward and cast cares aside, the more it shored us up emotionally. We left better equipped for the myriad of challenges we experienced in communicating. Our eyes had been opened to the fact we really *did* want the same things. We were refreshed in our resolve and our sense of being in this whole thing together.

We also came back that much more determined. Faith and time, sweat and perseverance would surely carry us. We just had to be patient.

Funny how different telling yourself that is from experiencing it...

Chapter Thirteen
Of Wayward Watermelons, Wichita Farewells, and a Wobbly Sense of Truth

While a new business found its birth, a school year was whizzing by to a rapid finish. I am still stunned when I think about how fast that first year went, especially in terms of the rich growth we saw.

Sarah and Timothy reached amazing heights—Timothy soaring in reading, participating and winning ribbons in his first math contest, and discovering cursive writing was so much easier on cramped hands, and Sarah blossoming in all subjects but especially striding ahead quite literally with her new physical therapist. He got her running and climbing when no one else could. And all without brooking nonsense or being overbearing.

My respect rose that much higher for this school district. There was nothing whatsoever wrong with the last one, but this smaller more intimate atmosphere had done so much more than we could've hoped.

And dear Elijah? Well, my oldest *did* struggle as only a preteen can, escalating a bit in argumentativeness and grappling more with the workload, but we also saw a startling passion for writing develop (complete with things he actually wrote down versus yarns unfolding in his head!), his first school dance endearingly attended, and a sense of responsibility begin to bloom like a rare flower springing from rough cement.

Or a watermelon where none was supposed to be.

Okay... I can tell that one needs explaining.

You see, spring and summer had seen us plunge into yet another new venture, one that both frightened and excited this thoroughly city girl—gardening.

I hadn't presumed to think about gardening at first, what with my black thumb and all, but a woman at church scolded me for my lack of faith, prayed with me for good results, and sent me on my way with the sense I might ought to give this whole growing thing a go after all.

It didn't take much to spark Joe, of course, or the kids with their sweet wonder of creation, and soon we were off and galloping. In our zeal, we snatched seeds left and right—cucumber and cantaloupe, peas and peppers, pumpkin and watermelon. Even flowers from marigolds to zinnias to sunflowers to my absolute favorite—morning glories.

Joe had staked out a large rectangular patch of the backyard just beyond my beloved clothesline where I did so much praying. Our adoptive Pretty Prairie mom and pop supplied some rich soil and encouragement, and, with a fair mix of apprehension and exhilaration, we set about scattering seed.

I spouted an awful lot of my unsure little prayers as I dug in that earth. A lot of "God help me...I don't know what I'm doing. Make it grow." Words that resonated far and wide—not just over a bunch of fruits and veggies but over our lives and times. I planted, watered, fussed, glanced often toward those airplane hangars behind us that whispered hopes and fears and wonders. We were over a year into this whole Pretty Prairie thing, and it was still difficult to see where it would all go.

And when cucumbers big as our forearms sprung up, I felt sure I knew exactly where it would go. But then when our lovely pumpkins and melons grew black and became bug fodder, I would lose heart again.

This garden...it followed the fluctuation of our times too closely to suit me. Joe had garnered a few more jobs, and somehow we always kept on. But there was a wanting tugging at me, a dark that kept coming along to shrivel the growth within and without.

Sunday trips to Wichita started becoming more than just a little strain. They were devastating to our pocketbook, and we were growing ever more unsettled in the sense of the church itself. I was still trying with all my might to keep a grip on the place that'd fostered me so lovingly through my single mother years, but something deep inside kept begging release.

Ironically, just as enthusiasm was cresting in those dear old walls, I was feeling all the earmarks of a crash and burn. I shrugged it off for a time as tiredness that would pass. Soon enough, I told myself, I would jump in the waves and feel all they were so obviously feeling. But the tiredness did not leave.

Summer saw us dry and striving to be saturated. We attempted to get to special services more often—pocketbook be hanged—in hopes to find ourselves filled. We read books, talked in hushed tones about the miracles, and unfurled bright banners of belief at the possibilities of seeing it all here and happening in Pretty Prairie, just the same way. We even volunteered in the children's classes, ready to give love and empowerment unto this next generation. Whatever that meant. I wasn't always sure, yet I was sure it just *had* to be good.

Still, reluctance persisted in me, and I berated myself for possibly resisting God. And then came discovery. And the shadow that had been in our midst longer than I cared to admit could no longer be ignored. I did research I'd never intended to begin. One word, one name piling upon another. Questions I'd long held in secret shame finding absolution. Exposure of much I had taken for granted yet punished myself for never fully possessing like the rest of them did.

And I saw, with a stab of pain like no other, that my beloved church family had begun following a man, chasing hype and unbiblical things, and it was not for us to remain nor subject our children to. Like a sweater, unraveled a thread at a time, much I'd been taught to hold dear to be truly Christian was coming undone at the seams. It was with an odd mix of sorrow and relief that I saw I was free. Though I'd only ever had the vague impression I was entangled, I was now free.

Forgive me if I don't detail every bit of it. It doesn't serve the purpose of this particular book or the health of my heart to defame others. I am not now—nor will I ever feign to be—a theologian. Just a shaky little sinner saved by grace looking to her Savior alone for answers, striving to attend to His voice for my every direction. One day, perhaps, when the pieces are better put together, I can clamber up onto that little soapbox with some measure of confidence...but not just now.

All I knew was that the joy we'd been fed over the years had turned to chalk on my tongue. And the answer to my every pleading, confused, and rather distressed prayer was a simple whisper:

This isn't real freedom. Move on.

We were on the cusp of digging into teaching in earnest, sorely in need of something miraculous to shore us up, and the answer was *Trust Me. Move on.*

It was with trembling hands and tear-rimmed eyes I worked at respectful but truthful letters to the pastor and children's pastor. I felt after they'd spent so many long and winding years guiding us, they were owed at least that much before we took our leave.

Error oughtn't bring despisement, I felt God say. Families remain families even when they must part in disagreement.

And that is the vein of what I wrote. To this day, I don't know how any of them really felt upon reading those words or whether it was dismissed to file thirteen as a head-shaking folly on our parts, caused hurt in their hearts, or stirred them to think.

As occasion would raise in me a wondering, I felt God clearly telling me time and again to let it rest. Let the blood cover it all. And if I struggled with any doubt, again and again, He was pleased to erase it for me.

It was odd, but we never even had to discuss where to go from there. Without a word, we knew that the dear church family who had extended so much—from VBS to warm prayers to the beautiful basement now outfitted with real walls the kids had gotten to play Van Gogh with—was to be our home.

It was different sinking into quieter pews after so many...shall we say... *lively* years. But I had gained perspective enough to see devotion wasn't dead just because there was order. Warmth abided in these walls in deeper and truer ways than my all-too-frequently empty arms had ever known.

Neither was wisdom restrained. There were dozens of chances to see that what God had revealed to me was also revealed to the teachers there—including the astounding day we walked into the Sunday School room to see several names I'd just researched right there on the dry erase board. The discussion that day was both enlightening and vindicating.

It was proof that the little old self-doubter—me—was, in fact, worthy of a word from God.

I felt like an eager puppy gulping up the bits offered. Joe had chances to expound in ways he'd not had before, and best of all, I saw the kids beginning to open up, participate, and understand. They found familiar friends they actually knew from school and enjoyed the structure I'd honestly feared might've chafed them after years of a much looser environment.

God's answer had been once again right under our feet all this time, waiting to be noticed.

Which circles back at last to that watermelon vine I referenced quite a while back... (Did you think I'd forgotten?)

As that summer began to wind down and a new school year readied itself, the garden out back had become a dense tangle, a testament to somewhat of a failure.

The cucumbers were long gone, and not a single fruit showed its face. Our few carrots were like something out of a cheesy sci-fi flick, peppers and peas were no-shows, and every last melon had long blackened and been devoured by birds and insects.

I'd chalked it up to my stumbly ways and had shrugged off thoughts of any future endeavors of the green thumb kind, sad but sure nothing but weeds would grow in this funky old place.

But then, one late summer night, Joe was out on the front porch enjoying the fresh air when he called me out to see something.

Crankily busy as per usual, I think I dropped my dishtowel with a fair bit of annoyance at being interrupted. "Whaaat?" I drew out the word in tired lets-get-this-over-with tones.

He simply said, "Look," and pointed toward the right side of the yard, just by the porch.

Curling away from the cement were some pretty, fairly good-sized leaves. I squinted. Familiar type leaves. A hint of a vine.

"Watermelon leaves," he announced wondrously, grinning like it was Publisher's Clearinghouse by his porch instead of a few leaves snaking away from it.

"Huh? How? Never planted any here." I shook my head, utterly dumbfounded.

Joe shrugged, and we considered the possibility of wind carrying seed clear from the backyard to this very spot by the porch. I didn't think so.

And then, like a sudden lightbulb moment, we recalled that first summer of leanness and simple pleasures. At one point, we had purchased watermelon. Sat out on the porch eating it fresh-sliced and ice-cold from the fridge. Joe had been teaching the kids the fine art of spitting seeds—something I confess had never crossed my mind once to teach.

I remembered my chuckled enjoyment at this utterly daddy-kid spectacle. Timothy and Sarah were fairly game—little Davey at not quite a year not old enough but fussing to try, of course, as with everything his siblings do. And Elijah?

Well, Elijah is a rather neat and rather OCD kid in many respects. Including spitting seeds. But as he so oft had begged over the years, he scooped up his little pile of black and asked if he could plant them.

Apartment-living years had always caused a regretful sort of "no" to be spoken. But that lovely summer twilight in our new rural surroundings? Sure, we thought with indulgent smiles. Why not?

The watermelon had been refrigerated for days. It'd never grow. But in the meantime, he'd have the fun of trying. And so we let him carefully scoop up earth, drop his precious bounty in, and close the dirt over it, arranging it neatly.

And naturally, we promptly forgot.

Until now, that is, one year later, staring at this sudden baby vine in our yard, right where he'd so tenderly planted!

I had to laugh. It was just so God! To cause the growth where He chose, when He chose.

And for *whom* He chose. Despite all reason, He'd chosen us for this little anomaly.

Expressly, *Elijah*, I believe, as a gift for his pure, untainted faith, and more as lesson for Joe and me to keep seeking after such faith.

Our eldest boy, a rare light of thrill shining in his sweet brown eyes, dutifully babied that vine as per our instructions. And just as fall was beginning to set in, a gigantic, beautifully striped watermelon expanded from that vine.

When Labor Day saw us with one of those few and prized opportunities to dip down south to my mom and dad's, we cut the miracle melon, as we dubbed it, taking proud photographs, naturally, and shared one of the sweetest feasts I dare say we have ever had.

Chapter Fourteen
How to Deal with Minor Crisis and Major Struggle Without Going (Completely) Round the Bend

That school year opened up in rather a scramble...and a lot of bugs.

Timothy had a project to begin tending to before the first day even commenced—twenty pictures of twenty different insects to be saved on a flash drive or something that could be transferred to the brand new iPads each student would be given for class. Because we did not possess the sort of modern technology that makes for crisp pictures or ways to save them as required, we'd spent the better part of those latter weeks of summer doing something that really had my mommy heebie-jeebies going full force.

We were taking baby food jars and scooping up every freaky little crawly thing we could find so he could transport them to school and *then* photograph them.

Luckily, with the sad old garden out back and a lot of open field behind us, the task proved easier than first expected. Timothy was a bit more the poised scientist/nature boy than I'd anticipated. And me? Well, I found myself a bit more able to tamp down the squirmy feelings inside than I'd thought I'd be.

Elijah was rather more quiet on the beginnings of his seventh-grade year. Very short reports on how it was to be switching classes more or on anything he was learning.

But there was little time to fret about it because it was at about this time that Sarah caught the dreaded head lice from a school friend. Talk about mommy heebie-jeebies! What made it worse was that she just couldn't shake them though we used every store-bought and home remedy known to man, did barrels full of laundry, and sprayed the dickens out of all that couldn't be washed to the point of near-paranoia.

We had tried to avoid that most drastic of scenarios—the short haircut—but between her missing her early days of school, the financial strain of expensive treatments, and the horror of combing, washing, and rewashing the hair of a frightened girl with a water phobia and an almost complete inability to be still, we bit the bullet and hacked away.

You must understand. She had always been known by her hair. Long, golden-brown, bouncy. So utterly girl, bedecked with ribbons and bows and sparkly ties. To go from that to her first pixie cut at the age of nearly nine was heart-wrenching for us both. Especially because I have little ability with the scissors. I took pictures and tried to soothe her by arranging it as best I could with her favorite princess crown barrettes, but her little face showed how she felt.

All I could do was hug her and reassure her it'd grow.

And between that and prescription shampoo, the nasty things finally died a certain death, so it was worth it in our eyes. And we reassured ourselves her cut was cute, easy to care for, and yes, it would grow.

Please, God, let it grow.

And if all that wasn't enough…

September saw other changes ushered in as well—ones that would show us yet again how God was orchestrating and providing those divine connections.

When we began attending the Mennonite congregation back in July, there was a very kind pastor. However, we had been told all along he was an interim, and there would be a permanent selection made shortly.

September introduced us to the new pastor and his wife. It was not long before we had a chance to sit down and have some very enriching conversations with them, as well as even lunch. There was much laughter, joking, and enjoyable game time.

They seemed neither stuffy nor unsure. Just warm, kind, and eager to bless Pretty Prairie. The pastor had an easy way about him, and I was pleased to discover his wife was well-versed in special needs, and the immediate kinship extended not just to Joe and me, but to our precious own as well, left me somehow unable to remain as guarded as I normally would.

I tried not to compare because it felt unkind, yet I could not help but note that although there were definitely times I felt a certain closeness at the old Wichita church, there was never this level of ease, and certainly never this personal feeling of value.

Maybe it was the small town setting that lent itself to really knowing each other, or the fact they were new, too, but as we launched into Wednesday night services—in this rural farming community, they run on harvest time, October to May, and just as in the old days, the boys of the family are still needed to pitch in— we had the sense this was not going to be any run-of-the-mill time.

For one thing, for the first time ever, Elijah was on his own steam, so to speak. In this little town, each youth group was terribly small on its own. So it was decided sixth grade and above would meet at the middle school under the covering of all of the churches. Thus, for the first time ever, he was attending in a different building than us and able to walk to and from on his own in good weather while the rest of us went to the big church and did our own things. He was shy about it all, but as was typical of him of late, he shrugged, said, "okay," and seemed willing to try.

And while I feared a feeling of separation, it was actually rather cool for each of us to have a place to go, from happy nursery time for Davey to classes for Sarah and myself, Timothy and Joe— who had the delight of plunging in to assist in our middle son's class and expound upon his rather deep Biblical thoughts and considerable experiences.

And meanwhile, I, surprisingly, found myself doing the same. We were doing a simple study of women in the Bible. I imagined most times I'd just slip into a seat and quietly listen and nod. Yet something in both the questions presented and the atmosphere had me sharing testimony like I'd never done before. I feared I was both a bore and a conversation hogger at times, but I discovered there was some measure of healing in it—both for me and for the ladies listening.

And pastor's dear wife became my biggest fan. She never shut me down, but rather, she encouraged my words. Thanked me. Considered them food for thought for those who perhaps had been a bit more sheltered in this small town life.

And for the first time in a long time, _I_ considered that, perhaps, I might just have something worth saying.

And so, it would seem, life had settled into a predictable, happy rhythm.

There were problems yet, of course. Money was tight, and Elijah was rather quiet and brooding—unless he wasn't. Sarah had her wobbly moments at school, and Timbo and Davey? Well, they were Timbo and Davey. Problems were few and far between there.

Timbo was eating up learning percussion and rolling along with other studies. Davey, in his second year, was delightfully blossoming into such a fun, smart, utterly charming kid.

My time was lending itself to a lot of wonderful one-on-one educating with my youngest. A lot of my best and brightest moments from teaching his age group came flooding back as I saw the possibilities. And he was and is such an eager student, seemingly unhampered thus far by anything—or refusing to be. Sometimes I think, like Timothy, he was born older.

So, suffice it to say, we were rolling along at a pretty decent clip, all things considered.

And of course, just as it usually happens when so much is so well…

Something came along to rock that rather glad little boat out of the water.

* * *

There really is no delicate way to say that there were discoveries made in this time about the three older kids, and especially Elijah and Sarah.

On a rather serene early November evening, it broke upon us like the proverbial bombshell in the course of rather ordinary conversation. Without distress, but in such a way it certainly could not be dismissed.

Forgive me that I, once again, choose sensitivity over detail, but suffice it to say, we were thrown. Utterly thrown.

This was the sort of loop-throwing that left us with little recourse but to reach beyond ourselves and seek the help of those we hoped would pray with us and give direction to our suddenly extremely shaky steps.

It is so tough as a parent to own up to the fact that maybe, just maybe, we'd missed some pertinent signs. Signs that emotions were more disturbed than we'd presumed. That our secure little world wasn't wrapped quite as tight as we had believed.

There was sick dread and questions and more sick dread and more questions.

It was hard to see the pain and the contriteness in the kids. I think we all wanted to make the problems go away and felt the heavy weight of being helpless to erase the past. Our family was more broken than it had appeared of late, and there was no way we could fix it on our own...not that we ever really could on our own. Jesus was and *is* needed first, last, and in between. Every hour, as the song goes.

And oh, did we need Him in *this* hour!

I feared taking the pastor and his wife into confidence even though I knew this was too big for just us. The idea of letting them see just how imperfect our family could be was heart-sinking. Though they'd been so very kind and so very friendly, I was almost sure that such glaring issues would be much too much when we'd really only just begun to know each other.

The welcome mat would surely be yanked away, distrust to take its place.

And yet, the compassion did not fail. The prayers were there to encompass us, the encouragement to seek what help was needed was readily given.

They believed in us yet. They believed in the *kids* yet. And such utterly Christlike behavior was humbling in its rare and unexpected qualities.

We shared with our parents and the school counselor as well and found ourselves met with that much more love and tenderness and prayer.

So...we moved forward, navigated some rather tricky business, and found ourselves linked with family therapists to address the needs.

It was not my first go-round with therapy, of course. I anticipated the prodding, the poking, the silent judgments. Like a garage sale customer picking through your pitiful display, looking for something of worth.

Guilt was an easy thing to reach for—like a hot, ugly sweater you don't enjoy wearing but put on because it's there. And boy, did I wear it.

I tried to shoot for upbeat but truthful, eager for help and recognizing the need for it. But I knew I must've reeked of self-consciousness and shame.

Joe, for his part, was, by turns, both taciturn and a wealth of information. Jokey to the point I knew he was uncomfortable, but still sincere about what we'd been up against.

We each had to strive to recall the honeymoon stage that followed our Marriage Encounter. This was where the communication rubber would definitely meet the rocky road. There were days I felt more up for it than others, honestly, and I venture to guess Joe felt the same.

Having to pull so much of yourself, your patterns, and your parenting skills out of the box to examine is never what I'd call something you are raring to do. The good of bringing it to light takes time to see.

The kids were as anticipated—Elijah cringed to discuss it all but knew the work ahead was necessary, Timothy was thoughtful and willing and very much my heart man, Sarah was giggly and gregarious as ever when faced with new adults to charm, Davey was happy and oblivious.

Underscoring all this, however, was a certain amount of apprehension at opening our doors and our hearts to someone new. Yet what we were met with was not at all the intimidating, condemning picture I'd envisioned.

Certain things needed to be addressed, yes, but we swiftly melted into friendship with these dear ladies, found ourselves affirmed again and again, and even had the opportunity to bear witness to all God had done for us. In turn, they began to outline some simple tools to increase peace at last. There was no one saying, "You're a bad parent," and there was not a single snide remark about anyone's weaknesses.

Just...love. And gratitude for how open our hearts were to receive. Yet another instance I could feel the hands of prayer lifting us higher than we could hope to climb.

And it didn't come at once, and we still have a way to go, but we actually really began to see growth—between the kids, between us, between the kids *and* us.

Bumpy starts and stops and restarts, to be sure, because honestly, there is no magical cure to relating with your family.

Just time. And grace. And more time. Adjusting expectations over here. Tweaking a word or two over there. Diffusing tempers and remembering to draw together in unity.

For my part, I began to see that as much as I longed to constantly step in and defend, there were times I had to withdraw and let Joe be Dad. There were days of finding more delicate ways to suggest instead of flying into full Mama Bear mode with paws swiping and growls erupting. A work-in-progress, naturally.

In addition to all this becoming a family, something else had to, unfortunately, find change and closure of sorts. When the children were adopted, visits to their biological dad were never forbidden. The stipulation had always been that the kids' well-being was never compromised.

These few and far between days of chilling with their blood father had long been met with a mix of gratitude and irritation— both for their randomness and his vastly different parenting style. Yet I don't know that I ever felt the strength within me to assert myself in this matter with the man who'd so powerfully wounded and subtly deceived me...

Until the light of so much discovery flooded forth, that is. Though I will certainly never be the sort of ex-wife to hurl blame in any old direction I please, it took me all these years to finally fully recognize that the visits were doing more harm than help. I think I always knew deep down, but that strong sense of longing for all to be right and well had superseded everything else for a long time.

Too long, I feared.

So…after a lot of prayer, the hard decision was made to suspend visits. The news was both given and met with a fair amount of sadness—for all intents and purposes, they still cared a great deal for him, his wife, and especially their half-brothers—but mixed in there was a surprising amount of resignation.

I can't say they understand on the level we as adults do, but somewhere in there is the comprehension he was a pretty fun person but not the man they needed him to be—and likely would never be.

To this day, emotions are still being sorted out, and the dialogue continues, but at long last, there was and is release. A freedom of sorts to move on.

And so…life rolled forward indeed. Thanksgiving and Christmas had again seen leanness in our pockets yet every need met—and then some, complete with an anonymous package with movie tickets for the whole troop. For the first time ever, we had a Christmas play to watch with all four of the children taking up parts—Timothy as Gabriel, Elijah the innkeeper, Sarah and David an angel and a star, respectively. I'd been almost afraid to expect such sweet providence and wonders to roll in yet again in our lack, yet He was and is so faithful. The way He delights to give good gifts to His children continues to astound me.

And then January broke in—a whole year of the business was upon us. It was especially hard, bitter, and unfriendly to the handyman. There were those few small, steady clients and amazing happenstances that somehow kept us afloat, but little that could be rightly labeled success. Even the government called us less than poor come tax time. Nothing to pay, nothing to get. A different sort of miracle, to be sure.

The school year marched forward—triumphs and setbacks abounded. There were days when emotions ran high but many more that saw great accomplishments—Timbo's percussion, Sarah's singing, and Elijah's creativity. And David just kept toddling along after them all, absorbing, chattering when it suited, and baffling us with all he could do—and wanted to do.

I think it has been both startling and a relief and to see him reach and exceed milestones with ease. I can admit to holding my breath a bit, looking for signs of autism or physical delay once more—as much as I'd never trade any of my beauties, and as much as I determined to always embrace all, come what may, I'd be lying to say I don't rejoice in David's present soundness. So much strength and, at times, heartrending work goes into a special needs parent's world...

As Elijah officially entered the realm of teendom, we saw some of this again. There were more than a few twists in his IEP this time around. It was decided more one-on-one time was needed to alleviate his tendency toward argument, essentially, but also because they could see his bright and lovely potential and would do anything to see it preserved rather than squashed.

It was a little deflating to see that after all these years of growing and learning, he needed more rather than less in the way of support. But it was rather gratifying to see the widespread love for this boy—from teachers to fellow students to therapists.

He also began therapy of his own, as well as, for the first time ever, having an official social group in which to practice those rather more daunting skills like conversation, turn-taking, and the like.

This seemed to quickly bring forth some good fruit. He was a little more animated, a little more willing to talk. Still very much a teen, mind you, but a little more at ease.

The crowning moment came toward the end of the year when the eighth graders unanimously voted for him to escort them off the stage at their graduation ceremony—a high honor, I was assured by his wonderful ally of an English teacher. In addition to this, he received a "Leader of the Pack" award for improved social skills, which truly thrilled all our hearts.

Timothy, for his part, continued to plow ahead in reading, honor roll, math. Perhaps a bit more emotional some days than others, and particularly articulate about his grief and confusion about all we'd been through in the past few months, but truly, forever and always my little rock, my funny goofball, and my insanely intelligent child.

Sarah saw many strides despite early struggles. Her independence and physical determination soared—the girl made it through the fifty and one-hundred-yard dash as well as a complicated obstacle course at her field day cheered on by a school full of fans. Her reading skills shot well above her age level, too. And of course, her joy, her songs, and her impromptu but startlingly rhythmic dances spread far and wide. Very, very little beyond the occasional dramatic whine intrudes upon her happiness. It is almost as though the whole growing up bit that has bogged Elijah down and caused Timothy some tears is something rather pretty and unfazing in her world—thus far, anyway. I must remember she is only just nine as I write this and keep ever before me one major truth I have learned in this old life and especially in the world of mothering autistics: never say never.

But oh, I hope to see her brightness never fade! To see any of their varied shades fade! What a glory that'd be—making every countless worrying hour so worth it all.

And so many times, I wish I could spend even just a single day seeing just like them. And I suppose, there are times I *can*—a least a little. When I sit down on the floor and spend some criss-cross-applesauce time just drinking them in.

Examining wicked awesome K'NEX creations that boggle the mind, watching drumsticks and imaginations fly, closing my eyes and letting the summer breeze of a sweet girl's song waft over me, joining in the little explorer's dig and bent for all things tool-related, just like Daddy.

Or just leaning back and eavesdropping on the colorful cacophony of their games, their unadulterated and utterly touching enjoyment of one another. Not that they are always squabble free, mind you. Far from it. But there is something so binding between them all that is so rare and something to behold.

Ah, you see—*that's* the miracle. Every bit as much as dividing lunch for the multitudes or placing spitballs in the eyes of the blind to give sight.

Please don't get me wrong here. Those are well and good and thrill my finite little mind upon reading them. Nor do I ever want to say such miracles cannot happen today.

I have had my comings and goings, excitement and misgivings in this regard, but the one thing I have learned is to never box in God.

He's unboxable.

But this...simplicity. *This* is a large piece of how He touches me. This is so often how He moves *me*.

Not in some grand show of power—though, dude, does He have it—or in some pot of gold twinkling with my name on it.

No, it's in the day to day, wow-this-is-cool kaleidoscope of angles I never dreamt of, and things I'd never witness if we were all so "typical."

It's in the purity of an icky, pooey, messy miracle He calls life— the life He gave me, the life I very nearly wasted, and the life I got back a hundredfold.

Chapter Fifteen
Greater Things Have Yet to Come

More should be said. Or so He tells me. So I'll listen.

Something you should know is…while all this goes on?

I find doubts in other areas today. As in *today* today. As I write it.

My little abuse survivor, frightened-girl-in-a shell areas. At times, I find these harder to keep at bay. There is that wrestling with worth, wondering when a breakthrough will burst in on the scene in full force, questioning if dreams deferred will find an absolution. Ever.

Questions of self don't just leave in the midst of being a mom, being a wife, or even being a Christian. They don't just vanish when the lights go on or forgiveness comes. I hope I don't burst any bubbles here, but…

Choosing to live for Christ doesn't equal a cakewalk. For anyone. I don't presume to be a special hard luck case. We all have something to survive. So no…no cakewalks here.

Some victories are more *cat*walk, in fact. Where some insecurities shake off, others cling. It isn't that you aren't really, really free in Christ…it's just that a whole new mind takes time to step out in, despite what you might have been told.

And my most leechy little insecurity?

Well, in the midst of striving to see Joe's and all my precious babes' dreams take flight, you see, I have been tiptoeing back to the arena of words I'd long abandoned in fear. Well, duh, you might say. I'm *reading* it. Ah, but you have no idea how long I have been grappling and dangling on this rope!

Ever since I could string words into phrases and phrases into stories, I longed to share them with whoever might have occasion to read. Yet like many young venturers of less than stalwart self-confidence, I swiftly folded under the sea of rejection letters. And then life took over quite handily thereafter, and time as well as inclination was rather unavailable for a good many years.

I even told God at several points I had nothing worth writing about. Go figure. He always provides, eh? :)

So anyway…when my heart began to stir again in earnest to put thoughts to paper, I was a bit paralyzed as to where to begin.

And then I began to browse on my phone, as that was the only Internet we could afford. And I read blog after blog. Beautiful stuff. Beautiful, scarred-up, messed-up lives salvaged by a most willing Savior.

Lives both like and unlike mine.

And suddenly, something seemed possible inside of me. Something begged to be told.

So despite our lack of Internet, I found a way to do a blog entirely via my little phone, and I began to pour forth.

Mostly communing with crickets and silence at first, of course. And then, ever so slowly, a voice or two chimed in. A couple even asking to pass my work on. And I began to ponder whether perhaps the story of this sad old gal might just have a healing property or two after all.

I began to send flurries of articles of all sorts for the first time in more than a decade. Where once I'd concentrated on coffee shop poetry and about a dozen failed starts at fiction, this time I just poured forth me—my survivals, my struggles, my view of autism through very nonclinical eyes.

I was literally swelling with the hope of possibilities…

And found myself face to face yet again with rejections. "Not our editorial needs at this time" kind of stuff. Canned but kind. As I write this, I haven't a single published article to my name. I know

I shouldn't admit to such. The writer's goal should be to puff up her accomplishments, but...

No. I am nothing if not completely real. Hope you've caught on to that.

So...a writer-in-half-bloom. Sounds better than wannabe, doesn't it?

And the funny thing is that that is where we sit at present on so many fronts. A life in the making, a house bursting yet with projects, a business in toddlerhood, a ministry but a word on our lips... (The airplane hangar I looked at on so many laundry days? It blew over in an early spring windstorm this year. Some even say it was a funnel cloud. Yet rather than that wiping out the dream, we felt God whisper to us, *It was just a clearing the way of sorts for the new.*)

Some might ask then, how do I know I even have merit? How do *any* of these stories have merit? They might even ponder what possesses me to write this *now*? Before they're grown? Before *any* of this is grown? While you still seem so much the "before" picture? While you're just...*waiting*?

No amazing ministry reports? No multi-million-dollar corporation? No alphabet soup behind your name to prove you really, really know what you're talking about? No raging Internet sensations or even a lousy leaflet with your name on it?

Just a ragtag family with a ragtag house and a lot of ragtag visions yet to be?

Well, it's quite simple really.

I warned this was no pep talk nor a list of magical keys to dealing with life. Not even a sermon since I'm not even a preacher.

But... (Yes, there is always a but.)

But...we have come *this* far in Him, with such amazing grace, it just *had* to be told, my friends. It wouldn't sit nicely in a corner waiting for my old age when my fingers would likely be too feeble to pound these keys.

For the message isn't how to be a success way down the road, or even how to be a success at all.

At least, not in the world's estimation.

If I have a message to all this madness, it's this:

Greater things have yet to come. Greater things are still to be done. This is only the beginning.

(Psst. If this was a movie, the above would be the broad wink to the audience to look for the sequel.)

But it isn't *our* greatness. It's *His*. It's both so timeless and so now.

In the now, live in *His* now. Don't look too far back, and don't strain too far ahead. Be well and be blessed right where you are. For *who* you are.

Autistic. Not autistic. Once abused. Abandoned. Divorced. Ex-felon. Mommy. Insecure. Klutzy. In crazy, happy second marriage-land, plugging away at something so very hard you just *know* it's so very worth it all.

Look for the unexpected, whoever you are and wherever you might be. Look for the miracle in the mess, the cross in your crossroads.

It may look broken, and it may even look weird. But it's there. And it's just as sweet. Trust me.

Made in the USA
Charleston, SC
16 July 2016